We Are Proud To Announce

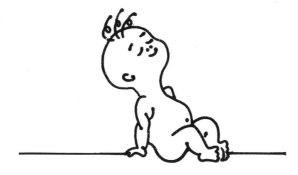

by

The Editors of Redbook Magazine

WALKER AND COMPANY **New York**

First published in book form in the United States of America in 1978 by the Walker Publishing Co., Inc.

Published simultaneously in Canada by Beaverbooks, Limited, Pickering, Ontario.

Library of Congress Catalog Card Number: 78:17629
ISBN: 0-8027-0617-7

PRINTED IN THE UNITED STATES OF AMERICA

Book designed by Lena Fong Hor

10 9 8 7 6 5 4 3 2 1

WE ARE PROUD TO ANNOUNCE

The wonder that makes every new-born child singularly individual inevitably inspires new parents to want to announce this special event in a special way. Mothers and fathers look for—and find—ingenious ways to announce the birth of *their* child.

This collection of prize-winning birth announcements and how to make them (with a bonus section on names and their meanings) is designed to spark the imagination of expectant parents everywhere. The sample announcements are from REDBOOK Magazine's popular "We Are Proud To Announce" feature that has brought hundreds of one-of-a-kind birth announcements each week for nearly thirty years. Many of them are inspired by name; the Grandys had a Baby Grand-y.

Occupations frequently spark an idea; auto dealers present a new model, publishers announce a new edition; avocations lead to sky-divers parachuting in a new arrival. Baseball pitchers fantasize they got a hit!

Some of the birth announcements REDBOOK has received over the years are professionally executed; architects and engineers frequently do detailed blueprints of their infants. Others are as simple as a pink feather attached to white note paper to say how tickled (pink, of course) they are to announce a baby's birth. Some are outrageously punny; Wendy Ann Cooley was a weather prediction. But all of them glow with the special incomparable joy that comes with announcing the arrival of a new baby.

May this book inspire your telling of your special joy.

Ruth Fairchild Pomeroy
and
The Editors of REDBOOK

Thank you

—to the nearly half million people who have shared their special birth announcements with us. We wish you could all have been winners.

—to the children, some still young, some now grown-up who are featured in these pages.

—to all of you who have asked for REDBOOK's help in preparing your announcements. Here it is.

Special thanks to Ida Danon Fidelman of the REDBOOK staff who has so carefully sorted through the mountains of mail addressed to "Department A" (We Are Proud To Announce) and first suggested that this collection of one-of-a-kind birth announcements be put in a little book.

Contents

"A Baby is God's opinion that the world should go on."

Carl Sandburg

Part 1

PROUD ANNOUNCEMENTS BASED ON NAMES

By all odds the favorite theme of individualized birth announcements is the use of the family name. Sometimes it's easy: The Warners announce a double feature, the Ushers give a front seat to their newborn and the Freys have a small fry. But it took some pondering for Mary Lou and Stephen Combs to ask that their announcement not be brushed aside, for the Winters to announce that the heaviest-yet (7 lbs, 12 ounces) had stormed in and the Geigers to ask Geiger counters to add one.

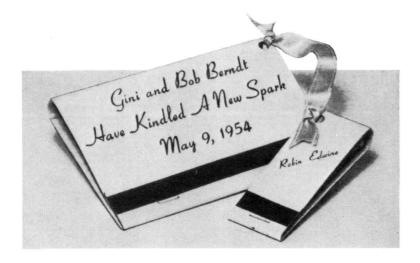

Although our family name is Berndt, it is pronounced "burnt," and it inspired my husband and me to try to devise an original card. These match folders are the theme which finally pleased us most.

Mrs. R.E. Berndt
Clifton, N.J.

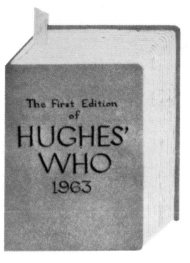

The First Edition
of
HUGHES'
WHO
1963

By hearing, rather than seeing their names the Hughes and the Coellns found original ways to say, respectively, "It's a boy; it's a girl." So did the Callenders with a heart marking the 25th of the calendar month of January as the birthdate of Richard Lance.

Kathleen Robbin
was born to
James and Kathleen Hughes
May 31 at 5:59 P.M.
in Laramie, Wyoming.
She was
21 inches long and
weighed 7 lbs. 3 ozs.

In announcing the birth of our first daughter, Kathleen Robbin, we decided to publish our own Who's Who. We called it "The First Edition" for our first child and used a pink bookmark for a girl.

Mrs. James Hughes
Midwest, Wyoming

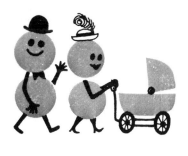

THE COELLNS
announce
a semi-coelln!

The Bairds stretched phonetics a little farther to announce that there were now "Three Bairds," and the Keyts gave flight to their imagination to announce that the Para-Keyts had a new fledgling. The Klocks signaled a time change; it was 3 o' Klock at their house.

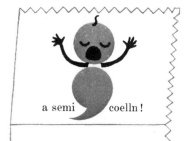

a semi   coelln!

Name: Lawrence Edward
Date: November 24, 1960
Weight: 7 lbs. 15½ oz.
Parents: Dick and Sandy Coelln

Despite the unusual spelling, the pronunciation of our name is the same as the word "colon." We decided to announce the birth of our first child, Lawrence Edward, by using punctuation terms.

MRS. RICHARD R. COELLN
Basking Ridge, New Jersey

9

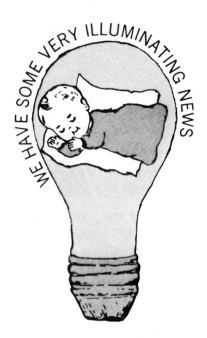

WE HAVE SOME VERY ILLUMINATING NEWS

The Watts and the Wagers were not content to produce illuminating news or a small wager. They did their homework on the appropriate language for their theme and came up with creative ways to convey the vital statistics of their newborns.

Mrs. William C. Watt
Mansfield, Ohio

Things are going to be much brighter around our house now, because we've just added another WATT!

The new "light of our lives" boasts these specifications...
BRAND NAME: Cheryl Lynn
PATENT DATE:
December 21, 1962
WATTAGE: 7 lbs. 8 ozs.
VOLTAGE: Girl   INCHES: 21
COMPANY PRODUCERS: Bill and Sharron Watt
ADDRESS: 222 Whittier Road, Mansfield, Ohio
MATERNAL GRANDPARENTS:
Mr. and Mrs. William A. Cousins
PATERNAL GRANDPARENTS:
Mr. and Mrs. William S. Watt

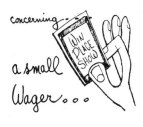

concerning...

a small Wager...

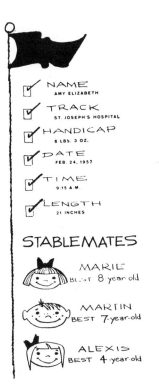

- ☑ NAME
  AMY ELIZABETH
- ☑ TRACK
  ST. JOSEPH'S HOSPITAL
- ☑ HANDICAP
  6 LBS. 3 OZ.
- ☑ DATE
  FEB. 24, 1957
- ☑ TIME
  9:15 A.M.
- ☑ LENGTH
  21 INCHES

STABLEMATES

MARIE
BEST 8 year-old

MARTIN
BEST 7-year-old

ALEXIS
BEST 4-year-old

We Won! and couldn't be happier...

ELLIOT   RITA

And the Fishers producing the Year's Best Catch recorded, of course, the weight and length but also gave the time and date of the strike, noted the species and named themselves as the anglers.

The descriptive tag that accompanied the little brick that announced the arrival of Douglas Edward Brick not only gave weights and measurements and delivery date; this superior brick was billed Durable • Washable • Won't Hold Moisture.

Here's the winning ticket, giving the results of our small Wager.

MR. AND MRS. ELLIOT WAGER
Denver, Colo.

THE CLUES

1. A CRY IN THE NIGHT

2. HURRYING FOOTSTEPS IN THE DARK

3. THE SMELL OF POWDER

"ELEMENTARY, MY DEAR WATSON."

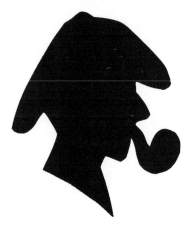

The Culprit: A new baby
The Crime: Stealing hearts
Born: August 19, 1975
            12:53 P.M.
Height: 21″
Weight: 7 lbs. 3 oz.
M.O.: Smiling, crying,
            being wet and cute
Accomplices: Katie & Jim Watson
Last Seen: 3596 Walnut Gr. Rd.
            Memphis, Tenn.

                    CHRISTOPHER
                    EVAN
                    WATSON

The Watsons obviously thought it no crime to designate Christopher Evan a culprit and the Katz found Andrew Simon a priceless pedigreed pet. Both families must have had a good time exploring every possible double entendre for their announcement themes.

The Henns hatched a little Henn and said so on the silhouette of a broken egg shell.

Since Jim and I are such murder-mystery buffs, we felt that this birth announcement would tell our friends of our "new arrival" and also show a little of our character. The materials were simple construction paper and paste.

KATHERINE P. WATSON
Memphis, Tennessee

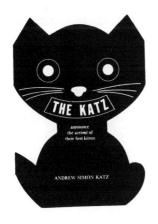

THE KATZ
announce
the arrival of
their first kitten

ANDREW SIMON KATZ

The Picketts, announcing the birth of their third child in less than four years declared they were building a Pickett Fence.

The Martins proclaimed the arrival of their first chirper and the Knights heralded "Lady Yvette" who "Mounted In" on March 8 of a leap year which provided not only an extra day but an extra Knight.

THE KATZ
ANNOUNCE THE ARRIVAL
OF THEIR FIRST KITTEN
ANDREW SIMON KATZ

The kitten's first meow was heard at Lynn Hospital on June 7, 1965, at 10:13 P.M. as the scales were tipped at 8 lbs. 13 oz.
Measuring 21" in length.
Pedigree papers were presented by Dr. Philip Snyder to Natalie and Loeb Katz.
This priceless pet is being groomed for showing at: 6 Arlyn Road Marblehead, Massachusetts.
Come purr with us.

Since our name "Katz" is pronounced properly as "Cats" and my husband sells animal health products, it seemed only natural to create a related item.

MRS. LOEB KATZ
Marblehead, Massachusetts

13

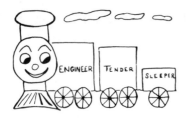

Our "Poehlmann"
Train has acquired a
New Little Sleeper!

While the Poehlmanns were anticipating a growing family, the Pecks used the arrival of their second child to turn their total into a bushel of fun.

When the Beers' third boy arrived they announced a new Short Beer—with Plenty of Kick.

engineer:
HARRY C. POEHLMANN
tender:
ELEANOR POEHLMANN
sleeper:
LISA KATHRYN
dimensions of new car:
18 INCHES
weight of new car:
5 POUNDS 12 OUNCES
initial run:
JANUARY 13, 1965

Although our name is of German origin, it is most commonly pronounced to sound very much like the word for the famous railway sleeping car, the Pullman. We decided to take advantage of this similarity to announce the arrival of our first baby. Now we hope that we will be able to use this same format several more times in the years to come, adding another "sleeping car" each time our family grows, ending, of course, with a caboose!

MRS. HARRY C. POEHLMANN
Monrovia, California

14

THE THREE PECKS

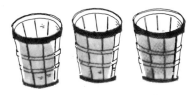

PROUDLY ANNOUNCE...
THEY HAVE BECOME
A BUSHEL

The Servis' declared they'd answered the call to "What This Country Needs Is A Little Friendly Servis."

The Beans greeted a little sprout and the Champagnes, after popping their corks with pride, allowed that Carole Jane, born two weeks late, was sweet, sparkling (if not dry) and added that internal aging had done no harm.

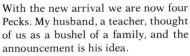

With the new arrival we are now four Pecks. My husband, a teacher, thought of us as a bushel of a family, and the announcement is his idea.

MRS. KARL C. PECK
Baltimore, Maryland

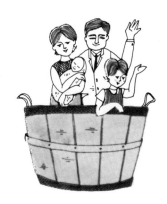

WITH THE ARRIVAL OF
KARL FRANCIS
ON MARCH 26, 1963

5 LB. 4 OZ.   18 IN.
WEIGHT   HEIGHT

WE'RE EXPECTING
TO HAVE A
FULL BUSHEL OF FUN.

15

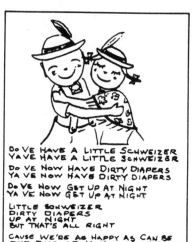

Do VE HAVE A LITTLE SCHWEIZER
YA VE HAVE A LITTLE SCHWEIZER

Do VE NOW HAVE DIRTY DIAPERS
YA VE NOW HAVE DIRTY DIAPERS

Do VE NOW GET UP AT NIGHT
YA VE NOW GET UP AT NIGHT

LITTLE SCHWEIZER
DIRTY DIAPERS
UP AT NIGHT
BUT THAT'S ALL RIGHT

CAUSE WE'RE AS HAPPY AS CAN BE
THAT TWO OF US NOW ARE THREE
J. SCHWEIZER

NAME - HEIDI MICHEL

ARRIVED AT. 12:31 A.M.

DATE - MARCH 25, 1974

WEIGHT- 7 lb 5½ oz.

PAPA UND MAMA- DENNIS & JUDY
SCHWEIZER

Ethnic origins swayed the Schweizers to song and the McNarys to welcome a wee bonnie lassie to the clan.

For the birth of our first child, we felt that with a German last name and the chosen name of Heidi for our daughter, an announcement with a touch of German would be most appropriate. Many of our friends and relatives told us how much they enjoyed its originality.

JUDY SCHWEIZER
Whittier, California

We've added to the Clan

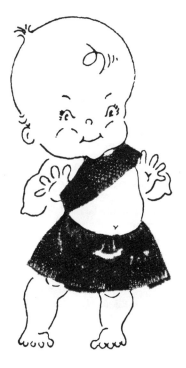

Joanne and Dick McArdle's announcement defined their twin girls' heritage: Kerry Anne (Kerry is Irish place name for County Kerry and Anne is German version of the Hebrew Hannah meaning "Grace") and Shannon Gay (Shannon is Irish place name for the River Shannon and Gay is Old High German for the beautiful and good).

My husband designed and made the announcements of the birth of our first child, Beth Elaine. Because of our Scottish heritage we wanted to announce appropriately the addition of our "wee bonnie lassie" to the clan.

MRS. KENNETH McNARY
Poughkeepsie, New York

our wee bonnie lassie

arrived March 1, 1960, in Poughkeepsie, N. Y., weighing one-half stone Jan and Ken McNary

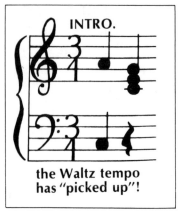

INTRO.

the Waltz tempo
has "picked up"!

with a daughter born in '59...
and a son in '61...the merry
Waltzes picked up their tempo
and had 2 instead of 1!

1st Musician	2nd Musician
Sarah Elizabeth	Susan Emilie
Entrance	Entrance
January 7, 1964	January 7, 1964
7:58 A.M.	7:59 A.M.
Weight	Weight
7 lbs. 1 ounce	5 lbs. 12 ounces
Length	Length
21 inches	20 inches

Conductor: TOM
Soloist: RUTH ANN

Twin arrivals prompted the Waltzes to pick up their tempo and the Budz rose bush produced two new Budz.

Bill and Jane Warner announced a world premier, their first Double Feature starring Demery Daher and Dana Martin with a cameo appearance by William Clay Warner, Jr.

Our last name being Waltz, we thought a musical theme would be quite appropriate for the birth announcement of our twins. We used the key signature showing three-quarter waltz time and the idea "we've picked up the tempo." Some friends of ours in our church run a printing company and printed them for us as a gift.

TOM AND RUTH ANN WALTZ
Elkhart, Indiana

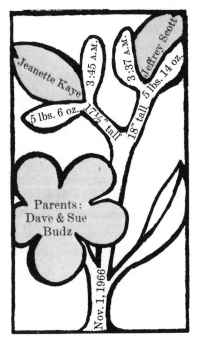

Jeanette Kaye
3:45 A.M.
5 lbs. 6 oz.
17½" tall

3:37 A.M.
Jeffrey Scott
5 lbs. 14 oz.
18" tall

Parents:
Dave & Sue
Budz

Nov. 1, 1966

Their announcement, like many, included the grandparents: Based on an original screenplay by the H.C. Warners and the G.W. Martins.

When the doctor informed us of our coming double event, naturally there were many last-minute preparations—the most important of which was the choosing of names! In one of the many books I found, there was the following passage: "Choose carefully. . . . A name like Rose Budd would be the subject of ridicule."

MRS. DAVID BUDZ
Peoria, Illinois

19

An ounce of Heaven
A twist of mirth
Filled to the brim
With this new Birth

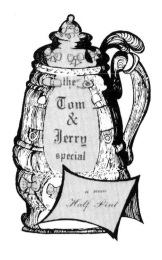

ANNOUNCING

Miss Tani Lynn Coleman

BORN

December 7, 1962

8 lbs. 1 oz.

PROPRIETORS

Tom and Jerry Coleman

Given first names often suggested an announcement theme. Tom and Jerry Coleman produced a new half pint.

The Shepards announced that Mary had a little lamb.

Dick and Jane Johnson, long the butt of jokes about Dick, Jane and Spot of the first-grade reading series, did name their puppy Spot. When their baby girl arrived, they were delighted to add a new character to "the never-ending saga."

To pass the long months of waiting more rapidly, we designed and printed the announcements of the birth of our daughter, Tani Lynn. We used our first names as the theme of the happy event.

MRS. THOMAS COLEMAN
Elizabeth, New Jersey

PROUD ANNOUNCEMENTS BASED

ON OCCUPATION

Adman, Mailman, Baseball player, Engineer, Lawyer, Jewelry maker—their life's work conjured up an image to translate into marvelous birth announcements. Jewelers produced a little gem, ice cream store owners added another scoop, grocers advertised mid-week specials and the owners of a mail order firm sent out a little first class male.

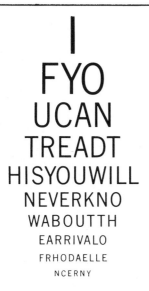

**I
FYO
UCAN
TREADT
HISYOUWILL
NEVERKNO
WABOUTTH
EARRIVALO
FRHODAELLE
NCERNY**

Announcing:
RHODA ELLEN CERNY
born
November 3, 1972
8 lbs. 12 ozs.
at
Memorial Hospital
Chapel Hill
North Carolina

My husband is an optometrist and thought up this way of announcing the birth of our first child, Rhoda Ellen. A friend printed the announcements on a home printer for us.

MR. AND MRS. JERRY CERNY
Durham, North Carolina

OUR RORSCHACH SHOWS

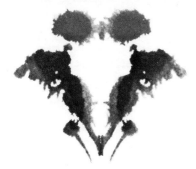

WE'RE CRAZY...
ABOUT BABIES!

David Edward Fluke
November 13, 1967
5 pounds 14½ ounces
1:58 P.M.

Psychologist Darrell Fluke and wife Joanne with two young children 15 months apart proclaimed with their third child that their Rorschach showed they were crazy—about babies. Advertising executive Terry Snyder recorded wife Lynn's true story in a familiar ad format.

The Chatterleys, perhaps resisting a romantic play on their name, opted to announce that their fifth boy gave them a basketball team of their own. Mr. Chatterley was the high school athletic coach.

My husband is working toward his master's degree in psychology at St. Cloud State College, and we decided to use the well-known Rorschach inkblot test as a device for our birth announcements.

The announcement took shape when a friend of ours remarked that either we must be crazy or we must love children, as our two youngest children are only 15 months apart.

MRS. DARRELL FLUKE
Moose Lake, Minnesota

22

My husband is an advertising executive, and to announce the arrival of our son we tried to think of an idea that would tie in with his profession. All our friends got a kick out of it.

MRS. LYNN SNYDER
Los Angeles, California

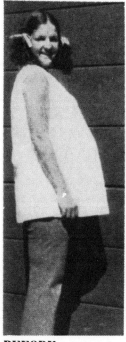

BEFORE

AFTER

How I lost 6lbs.,12oz. in only nine months!

A true story by Lynn Snyder as told to Terry Snyder

There I was, growing more and more each day. When would it ever stop? I kept buying larger clothes. Nothing would fit me any more. It got so I could hardly walk without waddling.

But then, on Sept. 6, 1972 at 9:14 p.m., a great thing happened. The growing stopped. My husband, who was with me at the time, as he was throughout the entire time, pointed, "Look," he cried, "A baby boy Let's call him Matthew Stephen Snyder, shall we?"

Of course, he was so adorable, we decided to keep him and now the three of us are living happily at 1140 S. Orlando Ave., Los Angeles, Calif. 90035 and I can once again walk in the sunshine, wearing my girl-like figure and chic outfits. The growing has stopped for me, but that little boy oh, when will it end?

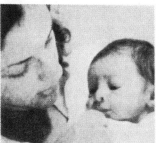

For more information on the life and times of Matthew Stephen Snyder, clip this coupon.

name: _____

address _____

city: _____ zip _____

phone: _____

☐ I'm interested in how this was done.
☐ I would like to know more.

23

Miniature mail bags matched father's occupation as a mail carrier and carried the arrival notice of the Richard Donlons' little boy. For the Catrons Mr. Zip had an extra-special delivery, twin girls Staci and Annie.

Men and women of the law took new arrivals into custody. Kelli Dalin Gull had been sought after for eight years by the Duane Gulls.

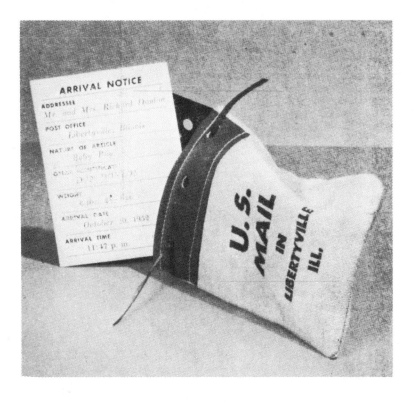

We wanted to produce a novel way of announcing the birth of our first child. Since my husband is a mail carrier, we tried to think of some connection with his job. One day he came home with the idea of the little mail sacks. We promptly went to work figuring out all the details of the announcement, and here is the result.

MRS. RICHARD DONLON
Libertyville, Illinois

An A.P.B. (All Points Bulletin) went out on Clint Wade Robinson known to arrive in Oklahoma City in the vicinity of Deaconess Hospital.

In Bellflower, California, Kristi May Brown alias "Button Nose" was taken into custody by Claire and Jim Brown. Subject's statement was recorded as "Loud Howling at Cruel World."

This announcement was designed and produced under the direction of my wife and myself to announce the birth of our second daughter. With such a lapse of time between our first and second child, we wanted something new and unique to make the announcement.

DUANE E. GULL
Castro Valley, California

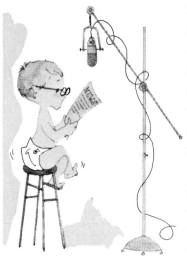

STATION WICK

PROUDLY ANNOUNCES AN
ADDITION TO OUR STAFF.

Stephen James III

ARRIVED ON *October 15th*
AT *5:06 pm*. HE IS
SMALL IN STATURE, ONLY
6 lb 8 oz BUT HIGHLY
QUALIFIED IN SOUND
EFFECTS AND SPOT
ANNOUNCEMENTS...

Communicators on the air waves chose symbols of their trade. Ruth and Stephen Wick announced an addition to the staff of **WMBI** in Chicago. He was highly qualified in sound effects and spot announcements.

Ray and Carol Andrews, both in television, used a roll-out teleprompter message with the news lead: 9 out of 10 doctors recommend babies to end long pregnancies. Their 6 lb. 15 oz. baby was named Marcy Lee for quick response.

My husband works at a radio station in Chicago. He is a producer/director and also does all the sound effects for the many dramatic programs WMBI airs. Therefore we used this theme to announce our little one's arrival.

RUTH A. WICK
Chicago, Illinois

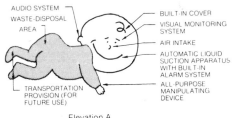

AUDIO SYSTEM
WASTE-DISPOSAL
AREA
BUILT-IN COVER
VISUAL MONITORING
SYSTEM
AIR INTAKE
AUTOMATIC LIQUID
SUCTION APPARATUS
WITH BUILT-IN
ALARM SYSTEM
ALL-PURPOSE
MANIPULATING
DEVICE
TRANSPORTATION
PROVISION (FOR
FUTURE USE)

Elevation A

Project: Baby Girl Number 1

Draftsmen, architects and engineers depicted their newborns in side, front and rear elevations.

The contractors were awarded bids with title, location and specifications spelled out. Contract limitations were included: 1. Noise abatement 2. Flood control 3. Multishift.

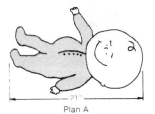

Alison Beth
June 20, 1976
7 pounds 8 ounces

Elevation B

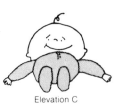

— 21" —

Plan A

Drawn by: J.H.
Checked By: S.H.
Scale: 21"

Hoffmann Design Group
Architects

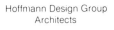

Elevation C

My husband is an architect, so we decided to fashion our birth announcement to look like an architectural blueprint. We think it came out rather well and that we'd like to share it with your readers.

Mrs. Susan Hoffmann
Hamden, Connecticut

Mr. & Mrs. Richard Osborn
eagerly announce a new
course of study
second semester . . .

Student-parents Marlene and Richard Osborn announced a new course of study: Richard Scott Osborn, Jr.

The Sid Martins put Susan Holland in a senior class with her father and awarded themselves in diploma-style MA and PA degrees from the U of P (University of Parenthood).

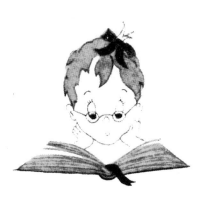

Registration for
their brand-new
assignment,
<u>Richard</u> <u>Scott</u>,
<u>Junior</u>, took
place <u>Feb. 18</u>,
<u>1969</u> at <u>2:10</u> <u>A.M.</u>
Although not a
heavy credit
load, <u>6</u> <u>lbs.</u> 13¾
<u>ozs.</u>, it promised
detailed home-
work and a
rewarding future
in the field.

My husband and I both are students at Wisconsin State University—Platteville, and since our baby arrived at the beginning of the second semester, this theme seemed fitting.

MRS. MARLENE OSBORN
Platteville, Wisconsin

The Wests and the Tituses anticipated army tradition to carry on when they labeled their babies "Chief of Staff" and candidate for "The Long Grey Line."

Food producers touted their new product. The Perlises, bakers in Bethlehem, Pennsylvania, inscribed doilies with realism: "It doesn't take a lot of crust but it sure takes a lot of dough—to produce Kenneth, moist, sweet and fully baked."

And from Young's Dairy Farm in Blakfort, Idaho, a new little squirt, Heath, who was Grade A.

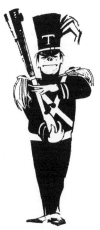

ANNOUNCING!
ANOTHER CANDIDATE
FOR
"THE LONG GREY LINE"
Arrival 0633 hrs.
Date May 2, 1961
Weight 8 lbs. 5 oz.
Name Ronald Carl
Parents Chuck and Peggy Titus

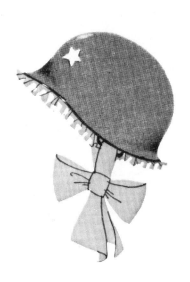

Having first gotten the idea of making our own announcements from REDBOOK, we proceeded from there. Since the first child tends to become "Chief of Staff" in any home, we thought this an appropriate way to announce the addition to our Army family.

MRS. MICHAEL F. WEST
Jolon, California

My husband, being an honor graduate of West Point and a career Army man, quite naturally was pleased that our first child was a boy. I designed and made this announcement to send to our Army friends. Now we are hoping our son will want to carry on the military tradition of the family.

MRS. CHARLES M. TITUS
Jacksonville, Florida

29

Telephone company employees invariably introduced an extension to their number or dialed a new tone or added a new party to their line. The Eliasons' triplets came in three models; the Kellys' charge/rate for their new subscriber was 4 ounces every 4 hours.

Additions took many forms. Nursery men grafted new stock (an adoption) on the family tree. Artists added a new color to their palette and carpenters added a new level to their tool chest. A shoe salesman produced a barefoot original.

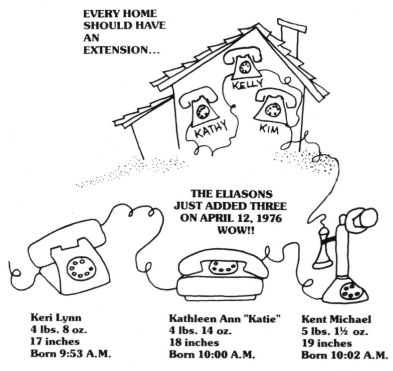

EVERY HOME SHOULD HAVE AN EXTENSION...

THE ELIASONS JUST ADDED THREE ON APRIL 12, 1976 WOW!!

Keri Lynn	Kathleen Ann "Katie"	Kent Michael
4 lbs. 8 oz.	4 lbs. 14 oz.	5 lbs. 1½ oz.
17 inches	18 inches	19 inches
Born 9:53 A.M.	Born 10:00 A.M.	Born 10:02 A.M.

When we discovered that the baby we were expecting was going to be triplets, we knew commercial announcements would be an impossibility. My husband is a marketing supervisor for the telephone company, so with the help of some co-workers he designed this telephone-related birth announcement.

KIM AND KATHY ELIASON
Lake Stevens, Washington

PROUD ANNOUNCEMENTS BASED

ON AVOCATIONS

Sometimes new parents felt their hobbies or some outstanding trait said most about them as a family. Scrabble enthusiasts spelled out vital statistics on a game board, crossword lovers solved a new puzzle and sailing enthusiasts announced a new arrival into port.

THE PUZZLE IS SOLVED

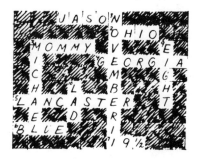

ACROSS

1. Baby's Name. ___ and the Golden Fleece.

2. Birth State. Home of the Buckeyes.

3. Baby Resembles. Not Daddy, but ___.

4. Mother. The Peach Tree State.

5. Town of Birth. A star of "Trapeze" was Burt ___.

6. Color of Eyes. The sky is ___.

7. Length. Halfway between 19 and 20.

DOWN

3. Father. Star of *Alfie,* ___ Caine.

8. Date of Birth. Veteran's Day.

9. Weight. Five and three are ___.

10. Sex. The opposite of lass.

As crossword-puzzle addicts, my husband and I felt it only appropriate to announce the birth of our son in crossword form. We got a big kick out of making them.

GEORGIA HART ALLERDING
Lancaster, Ohio

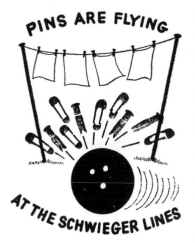

PINS ARE FLYING AT THE SCHWIEGER LINES

Bowlers and bird-watchers used the language of their sport. The Schwiegers announced they'd taken on the new job of pin-setting since the arrival of Dale Arlyn and the Drs. Pruess spotted a rare new fledgling, a persistent vocalizer that, they said, often sings at night.

Our son, Dale Arlyn, arrived shortly after the beginning of my husband's bowling season. As a tribute to his favorite sport, we carried out a bowling motif in our announcement indicating that we have taken on the new job of pin setting.

MRS. REINHARD SCHWIEGER
Fairmont, Minnesota

Letting you know we've
taken on the new job of
"pin setting"
since the arrival of—

Dale Arlyn
"sleeper"

Mr. & Mrs. Reinhard Schwieger
"pin setters"

10:32 A. M.   October 2, 1959
"strike"

19 in.   7 lbs.
"frame"

32

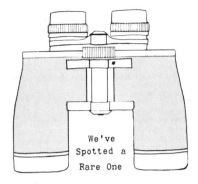

We've
Spotted a
Rare One

IT'S A FLEDGLING

Pruess extraordinariensis

Just out of the nest:

April 10, 1967
4:08 A.M.

Common name:
Carleen Elizabeth Pruess

FIELD MARKS
(female, juvenile plumage)

Weight: 5 lb. 11 oz.

Length: 19½ in.

Crest: dark, abundant

Epidermis: red and wrinkled

Habits: Persistent vocalizer,
often sings at night.
Frequently found in damp habitat.

Principal observers:
Dr. Kenneth Pruess
Dr. Neva Pruess

The Craters, avid gardeners, chose a seed packet to announce they'd developed a new hybrid, Scott Rainear. He was, naturally, a perennial that preferred a sunny, well-drained location and loving treatment.

I am an ardent bird watcher and so are many of our friends. It seemed appropriate to design our announcement in the form of a pair of binoculars, enclosing the news worded in ornithological terms.

MRS. KENNETH PRUESS
Lincoln, Nebraska

33

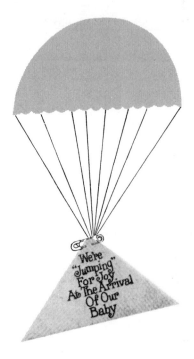

A sky-diving hobby inspired the Tony Bertones to announce they were Jumping for Joy at the arrival of Lisa Ann. The Ralph Basses, he an Air Force pilot, reported the safe and smooth landing of Carla Dee. They were heir-born.

My husband is an ex-paratrooper and his hobby is "sky diving." I designed our announcements and made them from one of his old parachutes.

MRS. TONY BERTONE
Fairport Harbor, Ohio

DATE
July 30, 1961
NAME
Lisa Ann
WEIGHT
7 lbs. 7 oz.
PARENTS
Judy and Tony Bertone

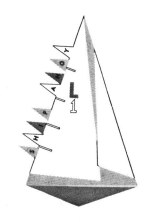

Sailing enthusiasts, Barbara and Russell Lenz recorded in the Lenz Log that a new shipmate was launched and christened Andrea Lee. From Honolulu, Skipper Abel August and First Mate Nell August signalled Michelle Ann's arrival into port. Her length was 20½ inches; displacement, 7 lbs. 6 oz.

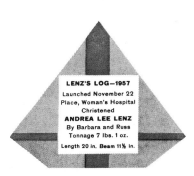

LENZ'S LOG—1957
Launched November 22
Place, Woman's Hospital
Christened
ANDREA LEE LENZ
By Barbara and Russ
Tonnage 7 lbs. 1 oz.
Length 20 in. Beam 11½ in.

To announce the addition of a new shipmate to our crew of two, we decided to use this sailing motif. Our friends know that our main interest in life is our 16-foot sloop, the Barbaruss. Now, we wanted them to know a new crew member would be handling the Barbaruss on the open waters.

Mr. and Mrs. Russell G. Lenz
Detroit, Michigan

Things to do:
1. paint baby's room
2. explain to Eric about birth
3. register for childbirth class
4. buy crib; layette
5. pick name; see separate list
6. explain to Eric about birth
7. pick route to hospital
8. go on hospital tour
9. make curtains
10. pack suitcase
11. explain to Eric...

12. design announcements

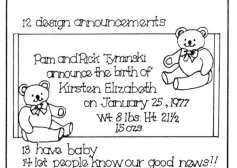

Pam and Rick Tyminski
announce the birth of
Kirsten Elizabeth
on January 25, 1977
Wt. 8 lbs. Ht. 21½
15 ozs.

13. have baby
14. let people know our good news!!

Pam Tyminski, known to her family and friends as an inveterate list maker sat down with her husband to list possible ideas for an original birth announcement. The result: a list that included their concern for first child, Eric.

In Tallahassee, Florida the Franceschis decided on the same technique. Theirs revealed that Gia Michelle was, surprise, not a boy.

Before the birth of our second child, my husband and I sat down together to list possible ideas for an original birth announcement that would in some way represent us. Soon we realized that we had our idea—a list! Our family and friends know that I'm always making lists, so one of them became the basis for our announcement, in which we also included our first child, Eric, by name. I hand-printed and designed one announcement and had copies made by a printer.

PAM UTTERBACK TYMINSKI
Columbia, Maryland

TALLAHASSEE MEMORIAL HOSPITAL
MATERNITY WAITING ROOM

Buy flowers for bail
Notify Internal Revenue Service ($625)
Design birth announcements
Call insurance man
Start college savings program
Write Vassar for application
  " Radcliffe " " "
Ask about diaper service
Get a 2nd mortgage on the house
Return cigars with blue wrappers
Return baseball glove and bat
Ditto football helmet
Collect bet from John
Ditto Sam
Pay off P.J.
Subscribe to Redbook magazine
See doctor about vasectomy
Library - get copy of "Promiscuity & Youth"
Check on child labor laws.

The Duane Franceschi's announce
Gia Michelle / 8 lbs. 13 ozs.
/ Friday, April 9, 1971

From Salina, Kansas Bev and Jerry Hedrick Jr. said things had been mighty busy around the Hedrick ranch since a new little cowgirl had joined them. Their list of "Things We Need to Do" included: making a new handtooled belt with the name Ginger Lorraine on it, pick out a pink saddle blanket and find a pair of Levis that will fit a 7 lb. 2 oz. cowgirl.

The idea for our birth announcement was mine, the execution by John Hanlon, Franceschi Advertising Incorporated art director.

DUANE FRANCESCHI
Tallahassee, Florida

The Basemans combined their name and his enthusiasm for sports to announce a third straight hit that loaded the bases. Their acquisition: a new bonus-baby, a third baseman.

Jane and Jim Beacham who "spend every spare dime on books" chose a book marker to say that their new arrival was one for the books. The authors of the new title, Jeanne Ellen, had waited 13 years for her publication.

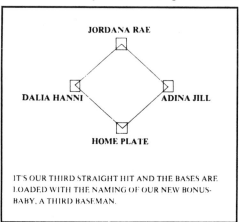

JORDANA RAE

DALIA HANNI   ADINA JILL

HOME PLATE

IT'S OUR THIRD STRAIGHT HIT AND THE BASES ARE LOADED WITH THE NAMING OF OUR NEW BONUS-BABY, A THIRD BASEMAN.

HER VITAL STATISTICS

Name	**AB** August Birthdate	**PCT** Performance Completion Time
DALIA HANNI	9TH	2:42 P.M.

HR Heaviness Recorded	**R** Range	**H** Hair
7 LBS. 3 OZS.	20 INCHES	LOTS

MANAGER .... RENEE BASEMAN
COACH .... ARTHUR BASEMAN
TEAM PHYSICIAN .... DR. ROBERT KELLER
PLAYER REPRESENTATIVES .. ADINA JILL BASEMAN
                            JORDANA RAE BASEMAN

My husband being such a sports enthusiast, and we being blessed with our third lovely daughter, we decided to take advantage of our surname. We reinterpreted some of the symbols utilized in reporting individual batting records to indicate Dalia's birth statistics.

Mrs. Renee L. Baseman
Clearwater, Florida

PROUD ANNOUNCEMENTS BASED ON LOCALE

Families far from home often chose symbols of the country where their child was born to send word to the folks back home.

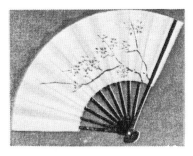

As frequently, state pride dictated the language and the pictures. The Georges who also admit to being a family of punsters from sunny California announced they'd been *Grant*ed a little *Ray* of *Son*shine (Grant Raymond George).

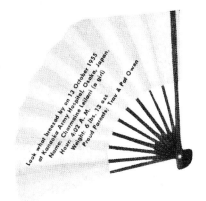

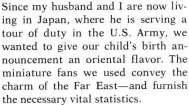

Since my husband and I are now living in Japan, where he is serving a tour of duty in the U.S. Army, we wanted to give our child's birth announcement an oriental flavor. The miniature fans we used convey the charm of the Far East—and furnish the necessary vital statistics.

MRS. TRAVIS OWEN
Osaka, Japan

From Germany John and Eileen Morrison sent word of the arrival of another tourist in picture postcard style. And Jean and Arnold Kluge chose a mascot of Australia to tell their relatives in California that John Arnold had hopped into being.

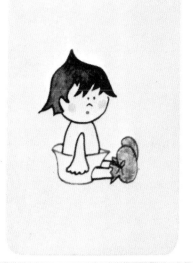

c/o The Morrisons
(John & Eileen)

Hi!

Just arrived in Europe. Having a wonderful time . . . . . . wish you were here!

Melissa Estelle

U.S. Boast Card

Redbook Editors

My husband and I have been avid tourists of the European countries throughout his three-year assignment in Germany while fulfilling his military commitment, so a picture post card announcing the arrival of another tourist seemed appropriate at the birth of our first child.

I typed the cards and prepared the rubber stamps used for the postmark and postage stamp with letters and numbers cut from discarded military stamps.

EILEEN MORRISON
Germany

TO JEAN AND
ARNOLD KLUGE
NOVEMBER 27, 1961
AT
KING EDWARD
MEMORIAL HOSPITAL
SUBIACO, W. A.
AUSTRALIA

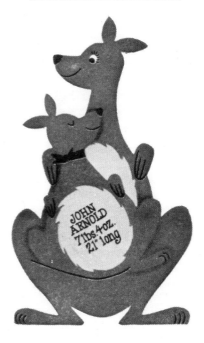

From France, Captain and Mrs. A.C. Willis announced the arrival of a little American in Paris. Monsieur Cigogne (Mr. Stork) delivered the news in French and English.

From Versailles the Abriouxes followed an old French custom, established by Louis XV of sending small boxes of dragees (sugar-coated almonds) to announce the arrival of Marie-Laure. The baby's name is inscribed on the box. These are custom made, pink for girls, blue for boys.

We are southern Californians living in Australia for a year while my husband is studying under a Fulbright Fellowship. Unable to find any birth announcements in the shops because Australians do not send them, we decided to make our own to announce to friends and relatives back home the arrival of our second child.

MRS. ARNOLD G. KLUGE
W. Perth
Western Australia
Australia

41

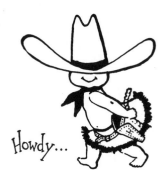

Howdy...

We have a new 'podner'

Name: Cynthia Anne Holt
Parents: Bill and Anne Holt
Date: July 13, 1957
Weight: 8 lbs.
Where: Houston, Texas

Few Texans can resist a mention of their state. The Holts of Houston announced that a pistol-packing "podner" had lassoed their hearts. Georgians sent their news in a nutshell. Philadelphians announced the arrival of a little Brotherly Love.

Our pistol-packing 'podner' has lassoed our hearts. Now she's napping, but soon she'll be roping all the hearts in Texas.

LT. AND MRS. WILLIAM T. HOLT, JR.
Houston, Texas

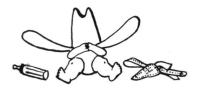

Mainite Pat Russell, and his wife Jan, used a sight of his childhood home to announce the birth of their "buoy."

Bill Erwin, then mayor of Flagstaff, Arizona, announced that he and Mrs. Erwin had fulfilled his Number One campaign promise: Planned Growth for Flagstaff.

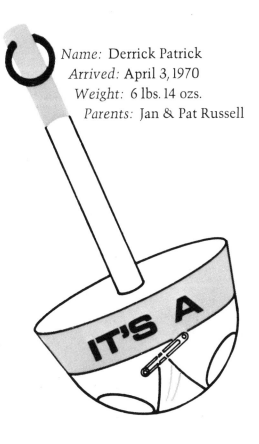

Name: Derrick Patrick
Arrived: April 3, 1970
Weight: 6 lbs. 14 ozs.
Parents: Jan & Pat Russell

My husband was raised in Maine, and since lobstering is well known in that state, he decided to incorporate the idea into our birth announcement. Thus the lobster "buoy."

An artist by profession, he designed and printed the announcement.

JANICE RUSSELL
West Newton, Massachusetts

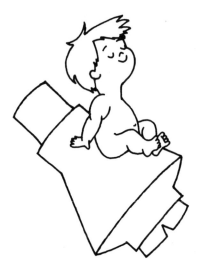

To celebrate the Seattle World's Fair, Bob and Phyllis Butler were the propellant forces that launched a new Seattle-ite. This was among the first of many space-orbiting announcements.

From Sharon, Pennsylvania the first Rose on the Hetrichs' family tree turned out to be John Paul, Jr.

We've launched a new
SEATTLE-ite

———

NAME: Erin Marie

TIME ENTERED ORBIT:
5:17 P.M.
August 31, 1962

PAYLOAD: 8 lbs. 2 oz.

SIZE: 19½ inches

PROPELLANT FORCES:
Bob and Phyllis Butler

———

Since our daughter was born during the Seattle World's Fair, Century 21, we decided to link the space theme with the name of our city in announcing her arrival. We called her our Seattle-ite.

MR. AND MRS. R.L. BUTLER
Seattle, Washington

PROUD ANNOUNCEMENTS BASED

ON FAMILIAR SIGHTS AND SOUNDS

A social security card, a hospital bill, a recipe, an income tax return—all familiar objects, all the inspiration for many prize winning announcements like the Mingos "playing" Bingo.

M	I	N	G	O
June	3	Ricki John	5 lb.	3 oz.
July	18	Cynthia Louise	7 lb.	5 oz.
Aug.	21	Robert Jon	12 lb.	6 oz.
Sept.	27	Cynthia Ann	6 lb.	9 oz.
May	30	Richard Robert	10 lb.	14 oz.

BOB & CAROL ANN MINGO
JUST MADE
BINGO!

Our name rhymes with the word "bingo," and that gave me an idea for our birth announcement. I used leftover thank-you cards from our wedding and drew the bingo card on the inside. For markers I cut circles from red cellophane. Since this is our first child, we included all the names we had chosen for him or her and used a red circle to mark "Robert Jon" on the card, which is the name we finally decided upon.

ROBERT AND CAROL ANN MINGO
Campbell, Ohio

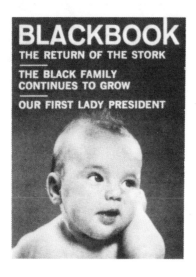

BLACKBOOK

THE RETURN OF THE STORK

THE BLACK FAMILY CONTINUES TO GROW

OUR FIRST LADY PRESIDENT

DR. GRADY COKER
Publisher

SISTER JEAN BAPTIST
General Manager

ADVERTISING MANAGERS
Dale and Donna Black

BLACKBOOK is published only once in a lifetime in the United States. President and Board of Directors consist of relatives of the new arrival. Executive and editorial offices: 716 E. Sixth, Concordia, Kansas.

Believing completely that imitation is the sincerest form of flattery, it's small wonder that the Blacks' Blackbook, a one-time-only publication, won a prize from the Editors of REDBOOK.

University professor John Cochran and his wife Mary granted a diploma to Jacquelyn Sue from the Universitas Obstetrica, upon completion of a prescribed nine months course. The degree granted: B.A.B.Y.

My husband and I have always been REDBOOK fans. When our second daughter was born, we wanted to adapt your format for our announcements. Using our name, we decided on the title Blackbook.

MRS. DALE BLACK
Concordia, Kansas

46

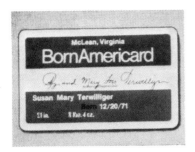

By her parents Roy and Mary Lou, Susan Mary Terwilliger was issued a BornAmericard to announce her arrival in McLean, Virginia.

In Winston-Salem, Edwin George Abel III became his parents social security and was issued a card to that effect which became his birth announcement.

With the advent of credit cards and the so-called checkless, cashless society, we thought this was a most appropriate and unique way to announce the birth of our daughter Susan Mary, since it ties in directly with my own field of finance and banking.

Roy W. Terwilliger
McLean, Virginia

Railroad man William Wieters and his wife Joyce announced that Celia Ann arrived on schedule.

The Mallorys of Austin, Texas had Deborah Kay on December 29th and delighted telling their friends, via an income tax return, that they had made the exemption deadline.

Military orders were the model for John Robert Nunay Monteith's arrival in a Marine Corps family. He was sworn in and accepted into the Monteith squadron and stationed, for the time being, at home.

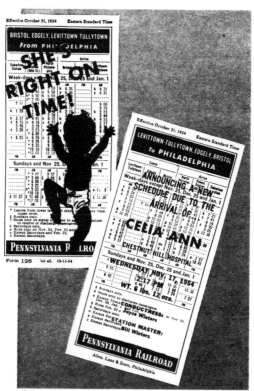

Since "proud Papa" works for the Pennsylvania Railroad, we decided to announce our new arrival with a timetable. Once we agreed we were on the right track, we had these copies made with the vital statistics superimposed. Celia Ann played right along with our train of thought by arriving on schedule.

MRS. WILLIAM C. WIETERS
Elkins Park, Pa.

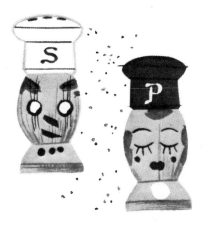

The William Bakers waxed poetic with their recipe for Bradley William, while the Gordon Bakers of Winnipeg, Canada provided a recipe for a new Cutie-Pie, Lynn Adele, perfected by her parents.

Shannon Renn Houston was billed as a recipe worth keeping: 6 lbs. 9½ oz. sugar, ½ cup artist (father Wayne). ½ cup teacher (mother Linda), 1 teaspoon ginger and lots of milk.

BAKERS' BATTER

Combine:

2 blue eyes
1 head of brown locks

Fold in gently:

7 lbs. 5 oz. of cuddliness

Add:

1 date—January 31, 1958

Yield: Bradley William

"THE BAKERS"—BILL AND BETTY

We announced our latest joy
(Our little Baker Boy)
With a recipe for batter
And (to simplify the matter)
A salt and pepper shaker

FROM BILL AND BETTY BAKER
Indianapolis, Indiana

Wednesday, September 2nd . . . Rainy Wednesday . . . About lunchtime there was this knock . . . Small fellow . . . about 5½ pounds . . . Maybe 21 inches head to toe . . . Built like steel . . . Determined looking . . . you know the type . . . Makes a point without bending . . . We were cautious . . . Stared at him . . . He stared right back . . . then, suddenly he snapped: "Where are the Dahls!" . . . We played it cautiously . . . "Who are you, Son?" "JEFFRY!" he proclaimed . . . "And I'm taking over as King Pin" . . . So that's the case . . . We're a captive audience . . . Dapper little diaper reigns supreme . . . Holds court daily . . . anytime after lunch . . . Remember . . . JEFFRY is the name . . . Another member of Guys and Dahls.

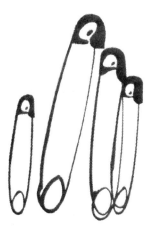

Mr. and Mrs. Joseph Norman Dahl
Clifton-Aldan, Pennsylvania

Tuned in to the stacatto speech of a familiar TV detective the Joseph Dahls recorded the arrival of Jeffry, another member of Guys and Dahls.

Representative David King and his wife Rosalie passed a House Resolution that their child should be known as Christopher Henry King, the eighth child of this family. The resolution was submitted by David S. King, member of Congress, Second District, Utah and carefully noted that "This was printed at the expense of the boy's father."

Whine List

Introducing our new house whine:

Briefly aged . . .
    dated
    October 21, 1969

Full-bodied . . .
    7 lbs. 9 oz.

Delicate feminine
    quality

Called
    "Sara Suzanne"

Very seldom dry

The whinemakers,
    Linda &
        Fred Crone

Vintners and other celebrants introduced a new blend or announced another vintage year.

Sara Suzanne Crone was briefly aged, full-bodied and very seldom dry. Other parents announced that their product would improve with age and reported a sparkling character.

This announcement was designed and produced by my wife and myself for the birth of our daughter. We mailed about 75 of them to friends and relatives.

FRED CRONE
San Diego, California

Paul and Jacque Schur announced a two for one stock split and guaranteed that all new shares were identical.

The Stoltes of Stratton, Nebraska issued a bank statement (new account) to Kathlyn Louise which asked "Please Examine At Once."

The Jimmy Isaacs of Chicago sent out an Accounts Receivable form (Mr. Isaacs is a CPA). Their Carol Jean was a new entry—in the pink.

THE SCHUR CORPORATION

ANNOUNCES A TWO FOR ONE STOCK SPLIT

Date of Issue: December 28, 1969

7:51 A.M.
7:55 A.M.

NEW SHARES: Jody Sheridan Schur
5 lbs. 13½ oz.

Jonna Sara Schur
5 lbs. 6½ oz.

(ALL NEW SHARES ARE IDENTICAL)

Corporate Officers

President Finance—Paul A. Schur
President Operations—Jacque S. Schur

My husband is a stockbroker, and our announcement was his idea.
Your "Proud to Announce" column is a real treat! We never miss it.
JACQUE SCHUR
Tarzana, California

52

PROUD ANNOUNCEMENTS BASED

ON SIBLING PARTICIPATION

Many parents, concerned with the anticipated problem of sibling rivalry, started with birth announcements to include an older child or older children. Here Jotham Herzon at age 3½ was encouraged to be the artist for his baby brother's announcement.

As an artist and jeweler myself, I have encouraged creativity in our first son from the time he was old enough to hold a pencil. When I told Jotty about the new brother or sister that would be arriving, he did a series of baby drawings (including "Baby with a diaper and diaper rash"). I decided to use one of them for our announcement, since I thought it would be a nice way for him to feel involved in the birth of the new baby—and I also wanted to do some bragging about our number one child as well as our number two.

SANDY HERZON
Albuquerque, N.M.

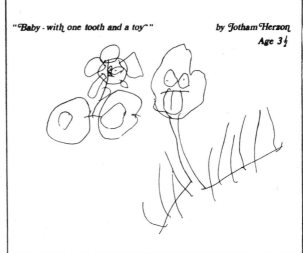

"*Baby - with one tooth and a toy* "   by *Jotham Herzon*
Age 3½

Baby Ian Everett
by Fred & Sandy Herzon

born Tues., April 9, 1974
time 4:35 am
wt. 8 lbs., 15 oz.
lgth. 22 in.

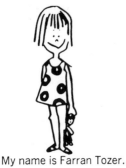

My name is Farran Tozer.

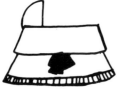

My mommy said that we were going to have an addition to our family.

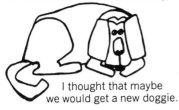

I thought that maybe we would get a new doggie.

Our baby—a girl
born May 24
—"KATIE"—
Katharine Coppins Tozer
6 pounds 15 ounces

Farran Tozer was among the many children who felt that a puppy would be a better family addition than a baby.

The Grundes wanted the birth announcement for their third child to tell everyone that her arrival was an experience celebrated by the entire family. Stick figures of the whole family drawn by the older children Tara and Mika announced baby Kathrina's birth.

Here is one of my baby announcements, announcing the arrival of our second little girl (I did the drawings).

My two-year-old is named Farran Tozer, and we thought that she should do the announcing!

I folded the yellow sheets and wrote the names and addresses on the outside, using staples to keep the paper closed.

Mrs. W. James Tozer, Jr.
New York, New York

Chopper Cheney issued the announcement of his sister's birth.

When the Basemans announced their third child the older children's names were on first and second base (see page 38).

When the Wagers announced their winning ticket, stable-mates Marcia, Martin and Alexis were also pictured (page 11). And the list-making Tyminskis (page 36) were as concerned with Eric as they were with the new baby.

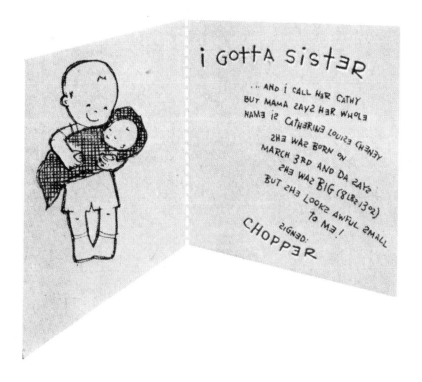

i GOttA sistɘR

··· AND i CALL HɘR CATHY BUT MAMA ƨAYƨ HɘR WHOLɘ NAMƨ iƨ CATHɘRINɘ LOUIƨɘ CHɘNɘY ƨHɘ WAƨ BORN oN MARCH 3RD AND DA ƨAYƨ ƨHɘ WAƨ BIG (8LBƨ I3oƨ) BUT ƨHɘ LOOKƨ AWFUL ƨMALL To Mɘ !

ƨIGNɘD: CHOPPɘR

To avoid any jealousy between our two-year-old boy and his new sister, Daddy just drew a picture of them both on the announcement. Chopper was thrilled to death.

Mrs. W.R. Cheney
San Francisco, California

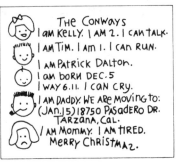

THE CONWAYS
I AM KELLY.
I AM 2. I CAN TALK.
I AM TIM.
I AM 1. I CAN RUN.
I AM PATRICK DALTON.
I AM BORN DEC. 5.
I WAY 6'11". I CAN CRY.
I AM DADDY.
WE ARE MOVING TO:
(JAN. 15TH)
18750 PASADERO DRIVE
TARZANA, CALIFORNIA
I AM MOMMY. I AM TIRED.
MERRY CHRISTMAS.

Tim Conway is known for his talent as a television actor but with the announcement of Patrick Dalton's arrival it's easy to expect Mr. Conway might have been a great efficiency expert. One small card included descriptive billing for Sister Kelly, Brother Tim, the baby Patrick, a new address, a tribute to Mommy Mary Anne and a Christmas wish.

Hope our birth announcement, change of address and Christmas greeting card can be printed in REDBOOK. My husband hand-prints it, then the printer makes a photo plate to run off a few hundred. Kelly and Timmy also had unusual birth announcements, but since they're over six months, you're unable to use them.

MARY ANNE CONWAY
Tarzana, California

P.S. Mr. Conway's talent and originality completely—I *just* have the babies! My husband is Tim Conway, co-star of "McHale's Navy," on ABC-TV . . . etc.

PROUD ANNOUNCEMENTS

BASED ON CURRENT EVENTS

When yet another remake of "A Star is Born" is released, the Stahrs, Starrs and Stars announce their babies' births with theater tickets, theater programs and posters proclaiming *their* star.

No continuing current event has inspired more announcements than the space program.

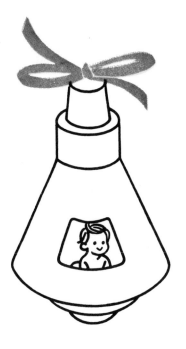

Successful recovery of a tiny space flier was achieved on February 25, 1962, by Mr. and Mrs. Robert F. Wallace. Initiated as Project I for the proud owners, Susan Lynn re-entered at a gross weight of 6 pounds and 6 ounces and measured 21 inches. The mission pilot will be maintained under careful surveillance for a number of years for debriefing and further training.

My husband is a public-affairs officer for the Project Mercury space program and works closely with the seven Astronauts. Since we were expecting our first baby about the time of Astronaut John Glenn's orbital flight, we planned our birth announcement with the wording in the form of a news release.

MRS. ROBERT F. WALLACE
Hampton, Virginia

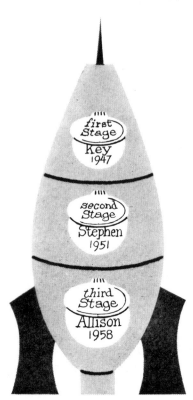

**ROBYN
ELIZABETH
Launched
into Orbit
May 12, 1961
Pay Load Weight
6 lbs. 8 oz.
Designing
Engineers
Hutch & Lucie
Stage**

The Stages elected to combine their name and news-making rocketry when they announced that Robyn Elizabeth was launched into orbit—the fourth Stage.

The Halbergs were excited about the arrival of the famous "Mona Lisa" in this country and pictured the painting on their birth announcement for Michele Kristen, their own masterpiece which left *them* smiling.

Our name brought to our minds the various stages of a guided missile. Having used the first, second and third stages for the names of our other children, we announced as the last stage the birth of our daughter, Robyn Elizabeth, on May 12.

Mrs. A.H. Stage
North Bend, Oregon

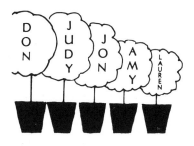

The Buschs joined in support of Lady Bird Johnson's "Keep America Beautiful" campaign by adding another Busch.

In Arizona Dr. J. Dale Nations, paleontologist at Northern Arizona University announced a new find previously unknown in his experience. He and his able colleague, Audrey, discovered a perfectly preserved specimen of a new variety of Homo sapiens while on their fourth expedition in search of it. The newspaper style story concluded with, "The rare and precious specimen may be observed along with many other objects of natural beauty in the Flagstaff area. Visitors welcome year round."

We tried to combine a reference to our last name in conjunction with our hobby of gardening.

And this is also a popular campaign of Mrs. Johnson's: "To keep America beautiful."

MRS. JUDITH BUSCH
Elkins Park, Pennsylvania

PROUD ANNOUNCEMENTS
BASED ON THE UNEXPECTED

WE KNEW···

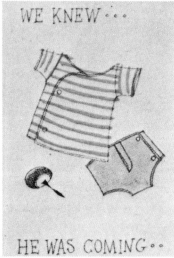

We were planning on a boy
To be our football Ace
But since it is a girl
It's football with lace!

HE WAS COMING··

It was exciting getting ready and making plans for the birth of the son we felt sure we were going to have. When we became the parents of a daughter we were very happy and made a number of changes to give her an appropriate welcome.

MRS. CHARLES BAXENDELL
Pitcairn, Pennsylvania

AND NOW SHE'S HERE!

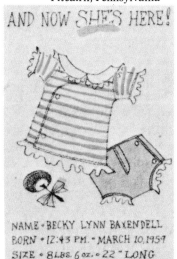

NAME · BECKY LYNN BAXENDELL
BORN · 12:43 P.M. · MARCH 10, 1959
SIZE · 8 LBS. 6 oz. · 22" LONG

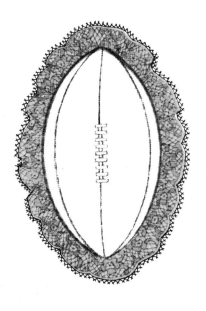

Name: Vicki LeAnn
Weight: 6 lb. 15 oz.
Date: November 13, 1959
Parents: Roy Lee and Ann
Black

PROUD ANNOUNCEMENTS
BASED ON JUST PLAIN FUN

Sometimes parents ignored their names, their professions and their home towns and simply pursued a thought that amused them and, they hoped, would amuse their friends.

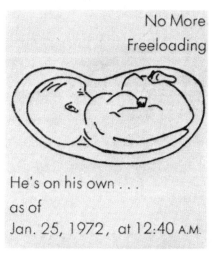

No More
Freeloading

He's on his own . . .
as of
Jan. 25, 1972, at 12:40 A.M.

"Freddy the Freeloader,"
now known as Erik Christian,
can no longer lie back and
depend completely on me
for life. At 21 inches and
7 lb. 12 ½ oz., Paul and I
don't think he'll have any
trouble.

Kristin Stadler

We referred to our unborn child as Freddy the Freeloader and thought it would be appropriate for our announcements. My sister, Carol Leerberg, printed the announcements for us.

MRS. PAUL W. STADLER
Enid, Oklahoma

61

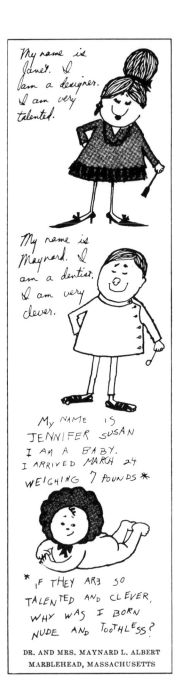

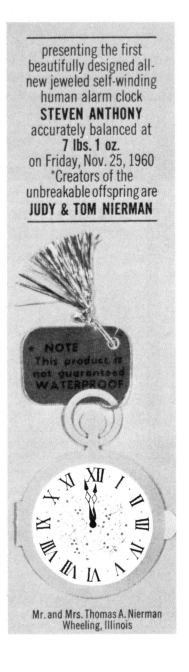

Part 2

WAYS AND MEANS AND UNUSUAL

MATERIALS FOR

MAKING ANNOUNCEMENTS

On the preceding pages you may have discovered inspiration for your own birth announcement. The next decision is how to go about making them. And that decision will depend largely on your talent and the time or money you want to spend.

By far the most common technique used in the selection of announcements was simple line art or photographs coupled with a handwritten or typed message. Duplicate copies of those announcements were usually made by a local printer.

If you are skilled in a particular craft such as silk-screening or photography, show it off in the execution of your announcements. But don't despair if you think you have no special talent and your budget dictates only an expenditure of time. There are several easy arts and crafts forms and do-able ideas that are effective and inexpensive and need not involve any commercial reproduction to make multiple copies. These are detailed on the following pages.

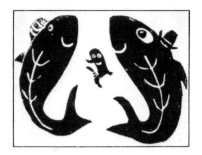

With the coming of our first child, we decided to take advantage of our name in designing our announcements. My husband is an art teacher and I am an artist, and we employed the linoleum print method in making them.

Mrs. James F. Bass
San Andreas, California

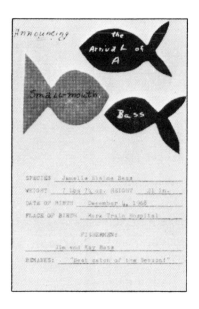

BLOCK PRINTING

The Basses used a linoleum block print to make their design and typed in the particulars of their announcement.

Block printing is an easy technique that uses either a linoleum block, a soft wood block or a potato. You make one design and print up as many as needed. Remember that in block printing your design will be reversed when it's printed. Note that Papa Bass is on the left of the block, on the right on the printed announcement.

LINOLEUM BLOCK PRINT

You'll need: Matte-finished paper, sized for the announcements; a linoleum block,* sized for your announcements; a set of small chisels, one small round gouge, one large round and one small V gouge*; an X-acto knife or a single-edged razor blade; a small rubber brayer or roller*; a piece of window glass; a soft-lead pencil, block-printing ink and plenty of newspaper and rags for cleanup.

STEP 1: Draw your design on paper; the sketch should be the size you want for your finished print.

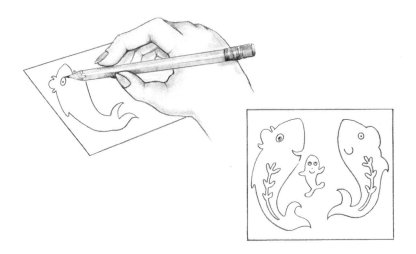

*Available in craft or hobby shops

STEP 2: With a pencil blacken the back of the design paper. Tape the paper blackened side down on the linoleum block and trace the design heavily so that it is transferred to the block.

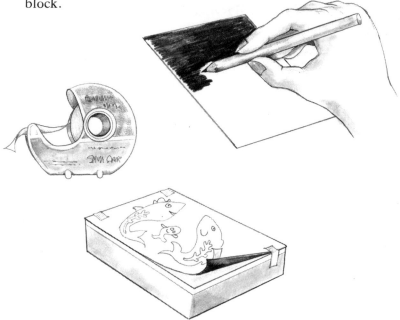

STEP 3: Using the chisels cut away the part of the surface you do not wish to print. Use the V gouge for fine lines, the X-acto knife or razor blade to smooth outlines.

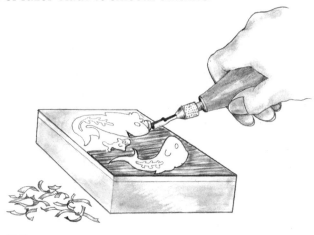

STEP 4: Squeeze out a small amount of block printing ink on the piece of glass and roll it with the brayer until it is satiny. Now roll the inked brayer over the clean, cut linoleum surface several times.

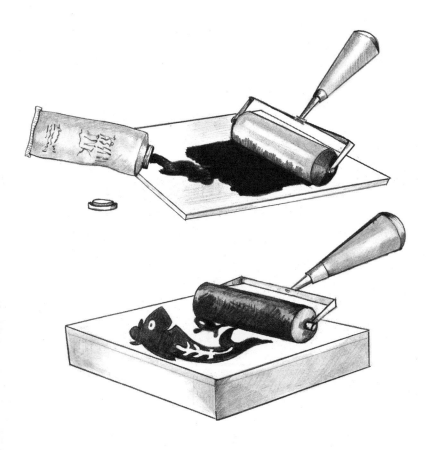

STEP 5: Pick up your printing paper by two upper corners, line the bottom up carefully with the block. Drop the paper down over the cut design (the ink will cause it to adhere). Rub over the paper carefully with the back of a tablespoon. Lift paper off and check results. If you have ragged edges or ink too thick or thin, now's the time to make corrections. If you're happy, continue to make additional prints.

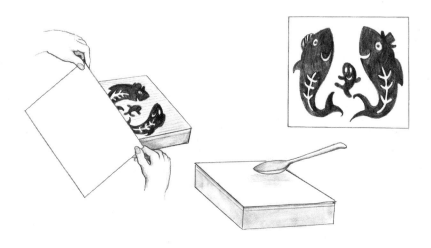

WOOD BLOCK PRINTS

Wood blocks are used in the same way as linoleum blocks. A soft wood, like sugar pine, is easiest to work with. Because of the grain, wood is a little more difficult to cut than linoleum. Original wood or linoleum blocks can be cleaned of ink or paint and washed with a color of your choice to use as a keepsake wall hanging.

POTATO PRINTS

Using a potato and a sharp kitchen knife you can achieve much the same effect as block printing with wood or linoleum, though the size of the design is limited. Wash a large potato and cut it in half smoothly. Sketch your design on see-through tracing paper and lay it face down on the cut surface of the potato. Cut around the design with a sharp knife, then cut away the part you don't want to print. For potato printing you must use water-based paints such as poster paints, tempera or water-colors. You can apply the paint with a brush or saturate a flat sponge with color and use it as you would a stamp pad. "Ink" the potato and press the

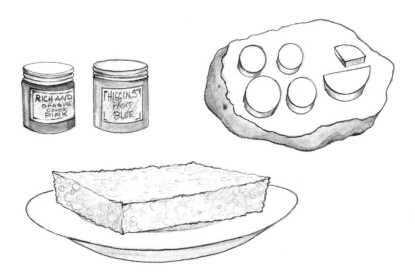

design directly onto the paper. The Coellns' announcement (page 9) would look much like this done in a potato print—the solid portions stamped out, the line features done with a felt marker.

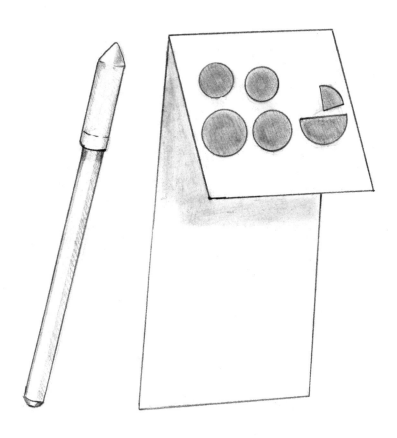

THUMB PRINT ART

This technique, used so effectively by the Rices to welcome a new "grain" to their field, is easy and not costly. Experiment with your design before you start on the final prints.

You'll need: A stamp pad in color of your choice;

a felt pen in color of your choice;

matte-finish paper.

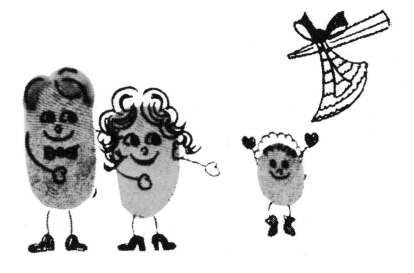

This Rice family has welcomed a new "grain" to their field!
Name: Angela Marie
Weight: 6 lbs. 1 oz.
Length: 19¼"
Date and Time of Harvesting:
March 11, 1975   5:38 p.m.
Parents: Jim and Elaine Rice

STEP 1: Roll your thumb firmly over a stamp pad and press the print in position on a piece of paper.

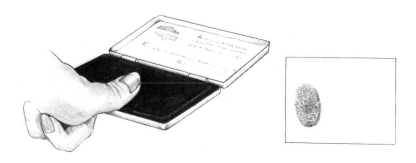

STEP 2: Add detail lines with a felt tip pen.

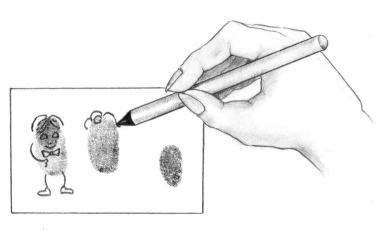

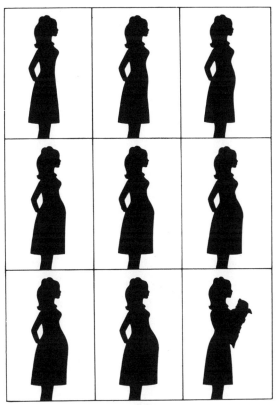

SILHOUETTES

Barrie Leigh Bernstein
July 24, 1973 8 lbs. 8 ozs.

Black-on-white silhouettes make an uncomplicated, clear design. The Watsons (page 12) used one in a simple style. In nine appropriate steps the Bernsteins told the story of Barrie Leigh's arrival.

Pasted-up cutouts from black construction paper (available in art stores) or sketches inked in with black india ink and a calligraphy pen that comes with assorted tips are the easiest materials to use.

Lack of art talent need not preclude using a silhouette. Stand your subject, or an object, between strong light and a sheet of graph paper taped to a wall and trace the shadow it casts. Graph paper allows you to reduce or enlarge the design.

PAPER CUTOUTS

The shapes of paper cutouts quickly convey an added idea for the announcement theme. The Lenz Log announcement (page 35) with cutout pennants flying is a perfect example. The only equipment needed is a steady hand and a cutting tool to match the weight of your paper. An X-acto knife used over a cardboard padding works well.

Professional advertising artist John O'Leary designed Mark's announcement that when cut out and folded, formed a child's building block. Mr. O'Leary silk-screened his design. It's a technique that produces beautiful results but requires special equipment and some skill. Crayons used on stiff paper could produce similar results. Note that block A (upper left) needs fold-down edges on three sides and April 1 block has folds on two sides. Tabs are on side of the BIG block and bottom of the April 1 block, *slotted* tabs at bottom of BIG block and side of MARK block.

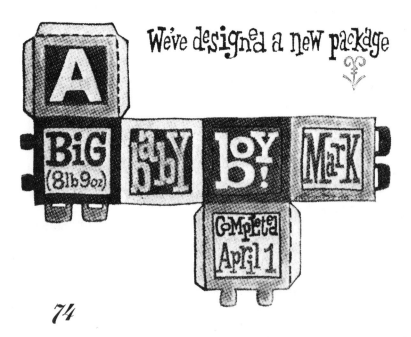

Black-on-white paper cutouts symbolized Rev. John Schrabel's calling. The black coat folded open to reveal a white T-shirt on which all the information about baby Timothy was written. An added filip: proud "popping" buttons mounted on foam rubber strips.

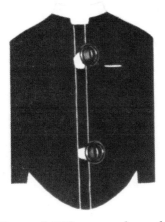

Susan and Howard Wilson used a white paper cutout bound at the fold with blue ribbon. Beautiful calligraphy script announced they now have a "handful."

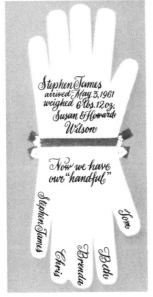

FABRICS, BUTTONS AND BOWS

The beauty of using fabrics, buttons, ribbons, rick rack is that, if sewing is a hobby, old scraps are likely to be on hand. Since these are time-consuming projects it's necessary to plan for either gender. Even then surprises can occur.

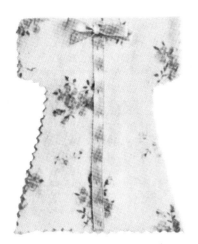

Mrs. Jerold Murphy's tiny flower-sprigged pinked-edged kimonos with a typed fill-in-the-blanks card enclosed was, in her words, "ruined." Son Scott arrived a month early which meant some last minute editing of the carefully typed message. Mrs. Bill Verdoorn solved the problem another way. She made up baby sacques in assorted colors and had two verses ready—one for boy, one for girl and cards were handwritten after the event.

Marilyn and John Workman designed a button and fabric-scrap announcement with inked in arms, legs and carriage details. The button-faced carriage occupant could have had an added curl if a girl.

When Dree Dublin arrived after two boys in the family her parents were prepared, hopefully, to add lace and patches of pink to blue overalls.

An all-purpose clear-drying glue and matte-finish paper work best for all fabric projects.

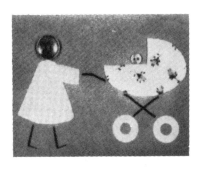

CUTE AS A BUTTON!

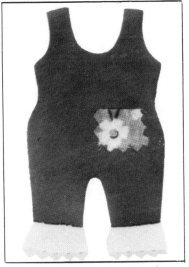

That's what Sara calls her living doll!
Name: Timothy John
Date: December 28, 1964
Weight: 8 lbs. 6 oz.
Parents:
Marilyn & John Workman

We're adding lace to hand-me-downs,
And snipping in the waist;
The patches are all made in pink,
Just to suit *her* taste.

INTRODUCING
Aundrea Alma Dahlen
Born August 10, 1964, at 11:31 A.M.
Height: 19 inches
Weight: 7 lbs. 2 oz.
Nickname: Dree
Hand-me-downs donated by
Greg & Jeff
Tailors: Avis & Jim
Visitors welcome to see model
and her wardrobe at:
1935 Verdugo Knolls Drive
Glendale

77

Avid sewers might tackle more ambitious projects like Susan Ann Harvey's miniature rompers for Patrick's announcement. Newspaperman-husband Paul printed the announcement on non-woven interfacing that slipped between the blue denim romper and the realistic plastic romper lining. The message could be written with fabric crayons or felt markers on the interfacing.

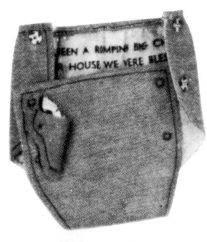

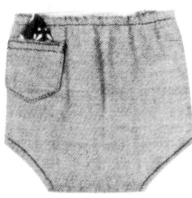

*There's been a romping
big change at our
house. We were blessed
with a darling baby boy.
We named him
Patrick Glenn Harvey.
He was born on
April 20, 1964, at 3:23 P.M.
He weighed 7 pounds,
10 ounces
and measured 20 inches.
And to spoil him in the
years to come,
his proud parents,
Paul and Susan Harvey*

PRINT ON FABRICS

Well before the popularity of printed T-shirts, the Gindis of Brooklyn, New York chose a motif to match Mr. Gindi's handkerchief manufacturing business. Their twin boys both bore the initials R.A.G. prompting quizzical remarks from their closest friends.

Other entries have included printing on diapers, miniature T-shirts and baby bonnets. When commercial printing is not available, fabric crayons or alphabet stencils would suffice.

The William Guthmans, in the clouds over William Scott's birth, had his announcement printed on large blue balloons.

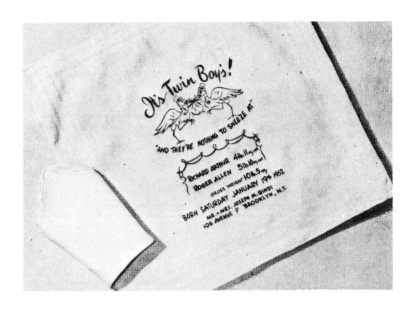

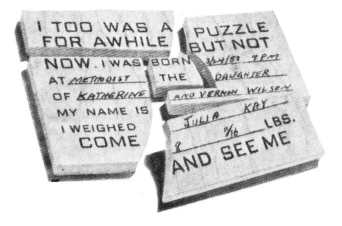

The Vernon Wilsons had a large stamp made, ready to add the vital statistics after Julie Kay was born. Mr. Wilson stamped the notice onto plywood and cut it into a jig-saw puzzle with a coping saw. Many other puzzle entries wrote their news on paper-covered cardboard which was cut out with an X-acto knife.

Ruth and Ben Hapner were ready with a spool of unexposed film that was printed in white ink and read: "After nine months of careful developing _____ has exposed herself to the world." Both the film and the puzzle announcements were sent in little mailing bags.

The Jacobs were ready and waiting to add Nanci Susan's name to their twine-rope ladder. And Mrs. Al Fisher had ready two shaped sheets of acetate in which to enclose appropriate felt cutouts to announce population increase in the "Fisher Bowl." A felt tip pen was used to ink in the birth date.

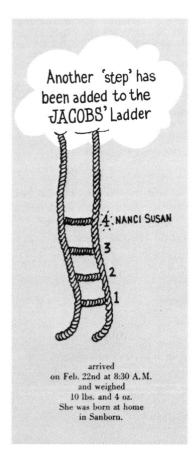

I couldn't resist using a fish theme to announce the birth of our first child. I glued pieces of orange, green and white felt to a piece of acetate shaped like a fish bowl and inked in the news of a population increase in the "Fisher Bowl." My husband then taped a second piece of acetate over the first.

Another 'step' has been added to the JACOBS' Ladder

4 NANCI SUSAN
3
2
1

arrived
on Feb. 22nd at 8:30 A.M.
and weighed
10 lbs. and 4 oz.
She was born at home
in Sanborn.

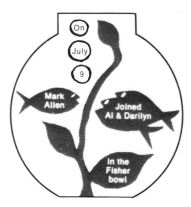

On
July
9

Mark Allen

Joined Al & Darilyn

In the Fisher bowl

Mr. and Mrs. Al Fisher
Flemington
New Jersey

81

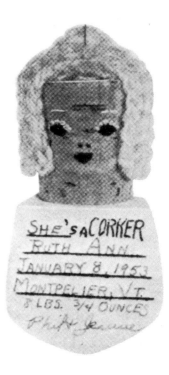

SHE's a CORKER
RUTH ANN
JANUARY 8, 195?
MONTPELIER, VT.
8 LBS. 3/4 OUNCE
Philip Jeanne

BUDGET-MINDED IDEAS

The Philip Corkers beat their pun-loving friends to it by announcing that Ruth Ann was indeed a CORKER. Scraps of yarn, drugstore corks, straight pins, a little paint, paper and glue were all that was needed to make a singular announcement.

The John Trottas remembered the similarity of expressions by a doctor using a tongue depressor and people viewing a new baby. They invited their friends to "Say Ahh" and inscribed all of Jonathan's statistics in red and blue childlike lettering on a wooden tongue depressor. Quick, easy, inexpensive.

By setting up the announcement on one side of a long sheet of paper, the blank side can be folded over, fastened with staples or a notary seal and used for addressing. This eliminates the need for envelopes.

The Nearings coated cut peanut shells with colorless nail polish, had a supply of pink or blue ribbons ready to tie in the typewritten news of David Anthony, Jr.'s birth.

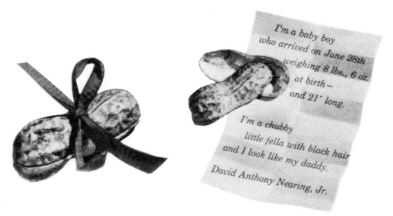

I'm a baby boy who arrived on June 28th weighing 8 lbs., 6 oz. at birth — and 21" long.

I'm a chubby little fella with black hair and I look like my daddy.

David Anthony Nearing, Jr.

Betsy Grunde's note with their announcement explained how they solved the expense of birth announcements.

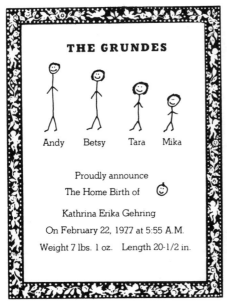

THE GRUNDES

Andy   Betsy   Tara   Mika

Proudly announce
The Home Birth of ☺

Kathrina Erika Gehring
On February 22, 1977 at 5:55 A.M.
Weight 7 lbs. 1 oz.   Length 20-1/2 in.

We wanted the birth announcement for our third child to tell everyone that her arrival was an experience celebrated by the entire family at home. Also it was important that the cost be kept to a minimum, because we had over 60 people to send them to and at the time of her birth my husband was unemployed. After some searching we finally found this stationery at the local five-and-ten. A typewriter, felt-tip pen and the amateur artwork of our older children did the rest.

BETSY GRUNDE
Sea Cliff, New York

83

Cigar-giving traditionalists found a way to lighten their announcements with humor. The Dosses' match packets were commercially printed. The Stefankos assembled their own sandwich men with a cigar and pipe cleaner arms and legs.

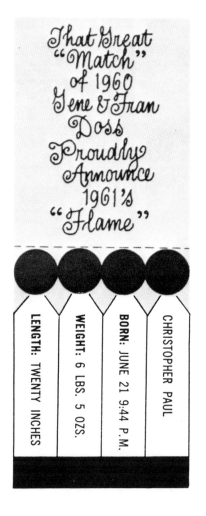

That Great "Match" of 1960 Gene & Fran Doss Proudly Announce 1961's "Flame"

LENGTH: TWENTY INCHES

WEIGHT: 6 LBS. 5 OZS.

BORN: JUNE 21 9:44 P.M.

CHRISTOPHER PAUL

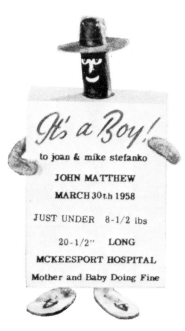

It's a Boy!

to joan & mike stefanko

JOHN MATTHEW

MARCH 30th 1958

JUST UNDER 8-1/2 lbs

20-1/2" LONG

MCKEESPORT HOSPITAL

Mother and Baby Doing Fine

Part 3

NAMES AND THEIR MEANINGS

"Must a name mean something?" Alice asked. "Of course it must," Humpty Dumpty replied. "My name means the shape I am." "With a name like yours, you might be any shape, almost," said Alice.[1]

Usually a baby has an assortment of names assigned to "him" or "her" before the ultimate day of arrival. There may be grandparents to please, friends to flatter, or parents may just like a given name.

Give thought to a child's name; it will be with him/her for life. Try repeating the given name with your surname to be sure it isn't a clumsy combination. Think about the initials formed by names. And try possible nicknames as well. Beatrice Minor may sound fine but Bea Minor may cause some titters in the first music class. While an unusual spelling of a name might appeal as truly individual, it will mean the bearer of it will be committed to spelling it out forever.

Names, both surname and given names all have an origin and a meaning. On these pages we've listed those given names most often submitted to REDBOOK's "We Are Proud To Announce" along with a brief description of their meaning.

1. *Through the Looking Glass* by Lewis Carroll.

Abbreviations used in listing

A	Arabic
Ar	Aramaic
AS	Anglo Saxon
C	Celtic
F	French
G	Gaelic
Ger	German
Gr	Greek
H	Hebrew
I	Irish
It	Italian
L	Latin
OE	Old English
OF	Old French
Sp	Spanish
T	Teutonic
W	Welsh

var.	variation
dim.	diminutive
f	feminine
m	masculine

Those names customarily used for girls are designated "f" and those for boys, "m." Given names currently used for either gender are marked "m,f."

AARON (H) (m)–High priest

ABIGAIL (H) (f)–Literally, my father is joy. dim. Abby, Abbie, Gail

ABRAHAM (H) (m)–Father; founder of the Hebrew race. dim. Abe

ADAM (H) (m)–Man of earth; mortal

ADELAIDE (T) (f)–Of noble birth or rank. var. Adaline, Adelina, Adeline. dim. Addie, Addy, Adela, Adele, Adéle (F)

ADRIAN (L) (m,f)–An Italian place name. var. (m) Adrien, (f) Adria, Adriana, Adriane, Adrienne

AGNES (Gr) (f)–Chaste, pure, meek. dim. Aggie

ALAN (C) (m)–Fair, comely. var. (m) Allan, Allen, (f) Alana, Alane, Alanda, Alanna, Alene, Alina, Allana

ALDEN (AS) (m)–Protector. var. Aldin

ALEXANDER (Gr) (m)–Defender of men. var. (f) Alexandra. dim. (m) Alex, (f) Alexa, Alix, (m,f) Sandy

ALICE (T) (f)–Truth. var. Alecia, Alicia, Alisa, Alyce, Alys, Alyssa, Allessia, Ellissa. dim. Allie, Ally

ALISON (T) (f)–Of sacred fame. var. Allison, Allyson, Alyson

ALROY (L) (m)–Royal. var. Alrey

AMANDA (L) (f)–Worthy to be loved. dim. Mandy

AMBER (A) (f)–A semi-precious jewel. var. Ambre

AMY (L) (f)–Beloved. var. Aimee, Ami, Amie

ANDREW (Gr) (m)–Strong, manly. var. (m) Andre, Andres, (f) Andrea, Andreana. dim. Andy

ANGELA (Gr) (f)–Lovely, angelic. var. Angelic, Angelica, Angelina

ANN, ANNA, ANNE (H) (f)–Derived from Hannah, meaning grace. dim. and var. Annie, Anetta, Anette, Anita, Nan, Nancy, Nanette, Nanny, Nina

ANTHONY (L) (m)–Worthy of praise. var. (m) Antony, (f) Antonia, Antoinette. dim. Tony

APRIL (f)–From the name of the month

ARNOLD (T) (m)–Mighty

ASHLEY (OE) (m,f)–One who lives in the ash-tree meadow

ARTHUR (W) (m)–Brave. dim. Art, Artie

AUGUST (L) (m)–Diminutive of Augustus, meaning majestic. var. (m) Augusta, (f) Augustine, Augustina, dim. Gus

BABETTE (F) (f)–A diminutive of Elizabeth

BARBARA (Gr) (f)–Foreign, a stranger. var. Barbra, dim. Bab, Babs

BARRY (I) (m,f)–Rampart dweller

BARTHOLOMEW (Ar) (m)–Plough man. dim. Bart

BARTON (OE) (m)–Barley farm dweller

BEATRICE (L) (f)–She who makes happy. var. Beetrix. dim. Bea, Bee, Trix, Trixie

BENNETT (L) (m)–A short form of Benedict, meaning blessed

BENJAMIN (H) (m)–Son of the right hand. dim. Ben

BERNARD (T) (m)–Bold as a bear. var. (m) Barnard. dim. Barney

BETH (H) (f)–House. var. Bethany

87

BLAIR (C) (m,f)–From the plain

BLAKE (OE) (m,f)–Black

BLOSSOM (f)–A modern name suggesting a flower

BLYTHE (AS) (f)–Glad or joyous

BRADEN (OE) (m)–From the broad valley. var. Bradford, Bradley. dim. Brad

BRADFORD (OE) (m)–From the broad ford

BRADLEY (OE) (m)–From the broad meadow

BRANDON (T) (m)–Dweller at the beacon. var. Brendon

BRENT (OE) (m,f)–From the steep hill

BRETT (C) (m)–One from Brittany

BRIAN (C) (m)–The strong. var. (m) Brian, Bryn, (f) Briane, Brianna

BRIDGET (C) (f)–The strong. var. Brigid, Brigette

BROCK (OE) (m)–The badger

BROOK, BROOKE (OE) (f)–Dweller by the stream. var. (m) Brooks

BRUCE (OE) (m,f)–From the surname

BYRAN (T) (m)–From the cottage. var. Byron

CAMERON (C) (m,f)–A Highland clan name. var. Camron

CAMILLA (L) (f)–A free born girl. var. Camille

CARA (C) (f)–Friend

CARL–See Charles. var. (f) Carla

CARMEN (Sp) (f)–Song

CAROLINE–Feminine of Charles var. Carolina, Carolyn. dim. Carrie, Cary, Karrie

CARTER (OE) (m)–Cart driver

CASSANDRA (Gr) (f)–A prophetess. dim. Casey, Cassie

CATHERINE (Gr) (f)–Pure. var. Caterina, Catharine; also Cathleen, Kathryn, Katrina, Kathleen. dim. Kate, Kathie, Kit, Trina

CHADWICK (OE) (m)–From the warrior's town. dim. Chad

CHAPMAN (AS) (m)–Merchant or trader

CHARLES (T) (m)–Strong, manly. var. (m) Carl, Carlo, Karl, (f) Charlotte, Charlene, Charline. dim. (m) Charlie, (f) Carry, Lotta, Lotty

CHERYL (Ger) (f)–Feminine of a German form of Charles. var. Sheryl

CHRISTIAN (G) (m)–Follower of Christ. var. (f) Christine, Christina, Christiane, Christiana

CHRISTOPHER (Gr) (m)–The bearer of Christ. dim. (m,f) Chris, Kit

CINTHIA (Gr) (f)–The moon. var. Cynthia

CLARA (L) (f)–Bright, illustrious. var. Claire, Clare. dim. Clarette

CLAYTON (T) (m)–From the town with the clay bed

CLIFFORD (OE) (m)–From the ford near the cliff. dim. Cliff

CLINTON (T) (m)–From the headland farm

COLIN (Gr) (m)–A diminutive of Nicholas, meaning people's victory. var. Collin

COLLEEN (I) (f)–Girl

CONSTANCE (L) (f)–Constant, devoted. var. Constantia. dim. Connie

CORBIN (L) (m)–The raven. var. (m,f) Corby

COREY (I) (m)–From the round hill. var. Cory, Korey

COURTNEY (f)–A modern girl's name, probably from the residence of Courtland

CRAIG (OE) (m)–Crag dweller

CRYSTAL (Gr) (f)–Pure

CURTIS (OF) (m)–Courteous. dim. Curt

DALE (T) (m)–From the dale

DAMON (Gr) (m)–Loyal friend

DANA (L) (m,f)–A Dane. var. (f) Danya

DANIEL (H) (m)–God is my judge. var. (m) Dannel, (f) Danette, Daniela, Danielle, Danile, Danila, Danita. dim. (m) Dan

DARCY (f)–A modern name possibly derived from Dara (H), meaning the heart of wisdom, or a diminutive of Dorothy

DARLENE (AS) (f)–Beloved. var. Darline

DARRELL (OE) (m)–Beloved. var. (m,f) Daryl

DAVID (H) (m)–Beloved one. var. (f) Davina. dim. (m) Dave, Davy

DAWN (AS) (f)–Day break or awakening

DEAN (OE) (m)–From the valley. var. Deane

DEBORAH (H) (f)–The bee, symbol of power. var. Debra

DENNIS (Gr) (m)–From the Greek God of wine, Dionysus. var. (m) Denis, (f)Denice, Denise, (m,f) Denys. dim. (f) Denette

DERIK (T) (m)–Form of Theodoric, which means ruler. var. (m) Derrick

DESMOND (AS) (m)–Protector

DIANA (L) (f)–Moon goddess. var. Diane, Dianne, Diann

DONALD (C) (m)–Dark stranger or lord. var. (m) Doran, Dorran, (f) Dona, Donalda, Donia, Donna. dim. (m) Don

DOUGLAS (C) (m)–From the dark stream. dim. Doug

DUSTIN (T) (m)–Valiant

DWIGHT (T) (m)–Fair

EARL (AS) (m)–Nobleman. var. Earle

EDWARD (AS) (m)–Rich guardian. var. (m) Edmond, Edmund, (f) Edmée, Edmonda, Edmunda. dim. (m) Ed, Ned, Ted, Teddy

EDWIN (AS) (m)–Valuable friend. var. (f) Edwina

ELAINE (Gr) (f)–Light. A form of Helen or Elena. var. Eileen, Ellen, Ellie

ELEANOR (Gr) (f)–Light. var. Eleanora. dim. Nell, Nelly, Lena

ELDRIDGE (AS) (m)–Wise counselor. var. Eldred, Eldrid

ELIZABETH (H) (f)–One consecrated to God. var. Elizabetta, Elsbeth, Eliza, Elise, Elsie. dim. Bess, Bessie, Betsey, Beth, Bettina, Bette, Betsy, Betty, Libby, Lisa

ELLIOT (OF) (m)–A form of Elias, Elihu and Elijah meaning Jehovah or God. var. (m) Eliot, Eliott, (f) Ellice

ELLIS (m,f)–A form of Elias, see Elliot

EMILY (L) (f)–Industrious. var. Emlyn

EMMA (T) (f)–Ancestress

ERIC (T) (m)–Powerful, kingly. var. (m) Erick, Erich, Erik, (f) Erica, Erika

ERIN (C) (f)–Girl from Ireland. var. Erina, Eren

ERNEST (T) (m)–Purposeful. var. (f) Erna, Ernesta, Ernestine

ESTHER (H) (f)–A star. dim. Essie, Hetty

ETHEL (T) (f)–Noble

EUGENE (Gr) (m)–Well born. var. (f) Eugenia. dim. Gene

EVE (H) (f)–Life

EVELYN (H) (f)–Derived from Eve. var. Evalina, Evaline, Eveleen

EVERETT (T) (m)–A form of Everard meaning strong or brave. var. Everet

EZRA (H) (m)–The helper

FAITH (L) (f)–Believing

FAWN (OF) (f)–A young deer. var. Faunia, Fawnia

FELICIA (L) (f)–Happy, fortunate. var. Felice, Felise, Felitia, Felita

FLOYD (C) (m)–The gray one

FORREST (AS) (m)–From the woodland

FRANCIS (T) (m)–Free. var. (f) Frances, Francesca, Francine.

dim. (m) Frank, (f) Fran, Fannie

FREDERICK (T) (m)–Peaceful ruler. var. (m) Frederic, (f) Frederica, Frederika. dim. (m) Fred, Freddy, Fritz, (f) Freddi, Freda, Frida, Fritzi, Fritzie

GABRIELLE (H)(f)–God is my strength. var. (m,f) Gabriel, (f) Gabriella, dim. Gabby

GAIL, GALE (OE) (m,f)–Gay and lively. var. (m,f) Gayle. dim. (f) Gay

GEORGE (Gr) (m)–Tiller of the soil. var. (f) Georgette, Georgia, Georgianna, Georgina

GLENN (G) (m)–One from the valley. var. (m) Glen, (f) Glenda

GORDON (OE) (m)–From the three-cornered hill

GRACE (L) (f)–Graceful

GRANT (L) (m)–Great

GRAYSON (OE) (m)–Son of a magistrate

GREGORY (Gr) (m)–Watchman

GRETA (L) (f)–A pearl

GRETCHEN (f)–Little pearl

HAROLD (T) (m)–Mighty in battle. dim. Hal, Harry

HARRIET (T) (f)–Mistress of the home. var. Hariette, Henrietta. dim. Hattie, Hatty

HARRY (m)–A diminutive of Henry or Harold

HEATHER (T) (f)–A flower name

HELEN (Gr) (f)–Light. var. Helena, Helene

HENRY (T) (m)–Ruler of private property. var. Henri

HILLARY (L) (f)–Cheerful. In modern use as a girl's name. var. Hilary, Hillery

HOLLY (T) (f)–From the holly thought to be a lucky shrub. var. Holli

HOWARD (T) (m)–Guardian

HOPE (OE) (f)–Literally, hope

IAN (H) (m)–God's gift. Variation of John

IDA (T) (f)–Happy

ILENE (f)–A modern spelling of Elaine. Also Isleen

IRENE (Gr) (f)–Peace

ISABELLE (f)–Considered to be a variation of Elizabeth. var. Isabel, Isobel, Isabella. dim. Bella, Belle

IVY (Gr) (f)–Sacred plant of Aphrodite. var. Iva, Ivey

JACOB (H) (m)–The supplanter. var. (m) Jaycob, Jacques, (f) Jacoba, Jakoba, Jacqueline, Jaclyn, Jocelyn. dim. (m) Jack, Jake, Jock, (f) Jackie

JAMES (H) (m)–A form of Jacob. var. (m,f)–Jaime, Jami, Jame. dim. Jimmy

JANE (H) (f)–See Johanna

JANELLE (f)–A variation of Jane. Also Ja-Nel, Janella, Janele

JANET (H) (f)–A diminutive of Jane. var. Janette, Janetta, Janice

JARED (H) (m)–The descender. var. (m,f) Jordan

JASON (Gr) (m)–The healer

JAY (OE) (m)–Quick, lively

JEAN (f)–A form of Jane. var. Jeanne

JEFFREY (T) (m)–A form of Godfrey, which means God's peace. var. Geoffrey

JENNIFER (C) (f)–White wave. var. Jenifer. dim. Jenny, Jenene, Jennee

JEREMY (H) (m)–A form of Jeremiah, which means appointed by the Lord. var. Jereme

JESSE (H) (m)–A gift of God. var. (m) Jessee, (f) Jessica, Jessie, Jessy. dim. Jess

JOAN (f)–Variation of Jane

JOEL (H) (m)–Jehovah is God

JOHANNA (H) (f)–God's gracious

gift. The feminine of John and the "mother" name of so many of the girls' names beginning with "J"–Jane, Jean, Joan and others

JOHN (H) (m)–God's gracious gift. var. Jon, Jan, Jean. dim. Jack

JONAS (H) (m)–A form of Jonah, meaning dove

JONATHAN (H) (m)–A variant of John. var. Johnathan

JOSEPH (H) (m)–Literally, he shall add. var. (f) Josephine. dim. (m) Joe, (f) Josie

JOSHUA (H) (m)–Whose salvation is the Lord. dim. Josh

JOYCE (OF) (f)–Joyful. var. Joy

JUDITH (H) (f)–Worthy of praise. dim. Judy, Jodi, Jody

JULIAN (L) (m)–A form of Julius, which means youthful. var. (f) Julia, Juliane, Julien, Julienne, Juliet. dim. (m,f) Julie

JUSTIN (L) (m,f)–The just. var. (m) Justace, (f) Justine

KAREN (Gr) (f)–See Katherine, var. Karon, Karyn

KARRIE (Gr) (f)–Variation of Carrie; a diminutive of Catherine. var. Kara, Kari

KATHERINE (Gr) (f)–Pure. A variation of Catherine. var. Kathryn, Katrina, Kathleen. dim. Kate, Kathie, Kathy, Kay

KELLY (m,f)–A surname used now as a given name. var. Keele, Kelli, Kellie, Kelley

KELSIE (f)–From the Norse Kelda meaning spring

KENNETH (C) (m)–Comely

KENT (C) (m)–Bright

KEVIN (C) (m)–Kind, gentle

KERRY (m,f)–An Irish county name. var. Keri

KIMBERLY (AS) (f)–In modern use as a girl's name. dim. Kim

KIRK (T) (m)–Church, one who lives by the church

KRISTINA (Gr) (f)–Variation of Christina meaning the Christian. var. Kristen, Kristi, Kristie, (m,f) Kristin

KRISTOPHER (m)–See Christopher

KURT (Ger) (m)–A form of Konrad, which means wise, able

LARA (L) (f)–A nymph

LARISA (L) (f)–Joyful. var. Larissa

LAURA (L) (f)–From the laurel, a symbol of victory. var. Laurel, Lauren, Loryn. dim. Laurie, Laurette, Lori, Loree

LAWRENCE (L) (m)–The laurel, victory. var. Laurence. dim. (m) Larry, (m,f) Laurie

LAYNE (f)–A variation of Elaine.

LEE (OE) (m,f)–Dweller in the meadow. var. (f) Leah, (m,f) Leigh

LESLIE (C) (m,f)–From the gray fort

LINDA (L) (f)–Diminutive of Belinda meaning beautiful

LINDSAY (T) (m,f)–From the island of serpents. var. (m,f) Lindsey, Lynsey. dim. (m,f) Lyn, Lynn

LISA (H) (f)–Diminutive of Elizabeth. var. Liza

LLOYD (C) (m)–Gray

LORRAINE (F) (f)–A place name

LOUIS (T) (m)–Famous in battle. var. (f) Louisa, Louise, (M) Lewis. dim. (f) Lisetta, Lois, (m,f) Lou

LUCAS (L) (m)–Light. var. Luke

LYNN (AS) (f)–A cascade. var. Lyn, Lynne

MALCOLM (C) (m)–Servant of the dove

MARC (L) (m)–A form of Marcus, meaning hammer. var. Mark, Mario

91

MARGARET (Gr) (f)–A pearl. var. Margarita, Margueretta, Marguerite, Margery, Marjory, Margo, Madge, Gretchen, Greta. dim. Maggie, Meg, Meta, Rita, Daisy, Mamie, Peggy

MARY (H) (f)–Original meaning is bitter but it is more commonly thought of as the name of the Virgin Mary. var. Mara, Maria, Marie, Marietta, Mariette, Marilyn, Marion, Marya, Mae, May, Moira, Molly, Moya, Polly

MARSHALL (OF) (m)–A marshal. var. Marshal

MARTHA (H) (f)–Mistress or housewife. dim. Marta

MARTIN (L) (m)–Warlike

MASON (T) (m)–A worker in stone

MATTHEW (H) (m)–Gift of God. var. Mathew

MAX (L) (m)–A short form of Maximilian, which means greatest

MEGAN (AS) (f)–Strong. var. Magan, Meagan, Meggen

MELANIE (Gr) (f)–Darkness. var. Melenie, Melyanie

MELISSA (Gr) (f)–Honey (the honey bee). var. Melise, Melisa

MELODIE (f)–A modern melodious name. var. Melody

MEREDITH (W) (m,f)–In modern use as a given name, probably from a surname

MICHAEL (H) (m,f)–Like the Lord. var. (m,f) Michel, (f) Michele, Michelle

MILES (L) (m)–Soldier. var. Myles

MILTON (OE) (m)–From the mill. dim. Milt

MOLLY (H) (f)–A variation of Mary

MONICA (H) (f)–A diminutive of Dominica, meaning belonging to the Lord

MORGAN (C) (m,f)–Born by the sea

MYRA (H) (f)–Wonderful. var. Mira, Mirilla, Myriah

NANCY (H) (f)–A diminutive of Hannah or Ann

NAOMI (H) (f)–Pleasant

NATALIE (L) (f)–A Christmas child. var. Natasha, Natoli. dim. Nettie, Netty

NATHANIEL (H) (m)–Gift of the Lord. var. Nathan. dim. Nat, Nate

NEAL (C) (m,f)–Chief. var. (m,f) Neil

NICHOLAS (Gr) (m)–The people's victory. var. (m) Nicholas, (f) Nichol, Nicole, Nicolette

NINA (f)–Diminutive of Ann

NOAH (H) (m)–Restful

NORA (G) (f)–Diminutive of Eleanor, meaning light. var. Nora

OBADIAH (H) (m)–Servant of the Lord

OLIVER (L) (m)–Olive, token of peace. var. (f) Olive, Olivia. dim. Ollie

PALMER (L) (m)–Palm bearer

PATRICK (L) (m)–Noble. var. (f) Patricia. dim. (m,f) Pat, Patty

PAUL (L) (m)–Little. var. (f) Paula, Paulette, Pauline

PETER (Gr) (m)–A rock. dim. Pete

PHILLIP (Gr) (m)–Lover of horses. var. (m) Philip, Phillipa, Piper. dim. (m,f) Phil

PIERCE (m)–A form of Peter. var. Pearce, Percy, Peirce

PORTER (L) (m)–Gate keeper

PRENTICE (L) (m)–A learner. var. Prentiss

QUENTIN (L) (m)–The fifth. dim. Quent

RACHEL (H) (f)–Ewe, which signifies gentleness. var. Rachelle, Richelle. dim. Rae, Ray

RANDALL (T) (m)–A form of Randolf, which means protector. var. Randal

RAYMOND (T) (m)–Mighty protector. var. Raymund. dim. Rae, Ray, Ramie

REBECCA (H) (f)–One who shares. var. Rebecha, Rebekah. dim. Becky, Reba

RENEE (L) (f)–Reborn. var. Ranee, Rene, Renne

RICHARD (T) (m)–Powerful ruler, dim. Rick, Dick

ROBERT (T) (m)–Shining fame. dim, Rob, Bob, Bobby (m,f) Robin, (f) Robyn, Robina

ROLAND (T) (m)–Fame of the land. var. Rowland, Roldan

RONALD (T) (m)–Mighty power

ROSE (L) (f)–A rose. var. Rosa, Roselle

ROSS (T) (m)–Horse

ROXANNE (F) (f)–Dawn of a new day. var. Roxana, Roxane

RUDULPH (T) (m)–Wolf. var. Rolf, Rolfe, Rollie, Rollo, Rolph, Dolph

RUTH (H) (f)–Friendly or beauteous

SABRINA (L) (f)–A legendary princess

SAMUEL (H) (m)–Asked of God. var. (f) Samantha dim. (m,f) Sam

SANDRA (Gr) (f)–A feminine diminutive of Alexander, which means helper of mankind. var. Sondra

SARA (H) (f)–Princess. var. Sarah. dim. Sally, Sadie

SCOTT (OE) (m)–A Scotsman. var. Scot

SETH (H) (m)–The appointed

SHANNON (f)–An Irish place name

SHEILA)f)–Irish form of Cecilia, which commemorates St. Cecilia. var. Sheelah

SIBYL (Gr) (f)–Wise. var. Sybil

SOPHIA (Gr) (f)–Wisdom. var. Sonia, Sonya, Sophie

STACEY (L) (f)–Stable or dependable. var. Staci, Stacy

STANLEY (OE) (m)–A form of Stanislaus, meaning glory. dim. Stan

STEPHEN (Gr) (m)–A crown. var. (m) Steven, Stefan, (f) Stefanie, Stephanie. dim. Steve

STUART (AS) (m)–A steward. var. Stewart

SUSAN (H) (f)–Lily. var. Susannah, Susanne, Susanna. dim. Sue, Susie

SYLVIA (L) (f)–Forest maiden. var. Silvia

TAMARA (H) (f)–Palm tree. dim. Tammy

TARA (G) (f)–Tower. var. Tarin

THEODORE (Gr) (m)–Divine gift. dim. Ted, Teddy, Terry

THERESA (L) (f)–Reaper. var. Therese. dim. Teri, Terry, Tess, Tessa

THOMAS (H) (m)–The twin. var. (f) Thomassina, dim. (m,f) Tommy

THORNE (OE) (m)–A form of Thornton, which means from the thorn tree

TIFFANY (f)–Probably from a surname. var. Tifany, Tiffanie

TIMOTHY (Gr) (m)–In honor of God. dim. Tim

TOBIN (H) (m)–A form of Tobias, which means goodness of the Lord

TRACY (AS) (m,f)–Courageous. var. (m,f) Tracey, (f) Traci, Tracie

TRAVIS (OF) (m)–From the cross road. var. Travers

TREVOR (c) (m)–Prudent

TYLER (OE) (m)–Maker of bricks

URSULA (Gr) (f)–Derived from the Greek nymph Ursa

93

VALERIE (L) (f)–Valorous
VANESSA (Gr) (f)–Butterfly
VERONICA (L) (f)–A diminutive of
Verna, which means born in the
Spring
VICTORIA (L) (f)–Victorious. dim.
Vicki, Vicky
VINCENT (L) (m)–Conquering.
dim. Vin, Vinn
VIRGINIA (L) (f)–Maidenly,
virginal. dim. Ginni, Ginny

Wainright, which means wagon
maker
WHEELER (OE) (m)–From the
surname
WHITNEY (AS) (m,f)–From the
white island
WILLIAM (T) (m)–Great protector.
var. (m) Wilhelm, (f) Wilhel-
mina. dim. Will, Bill, Billy, (f)
Willa, Willette, Billie
WILTON (OE) (m)–From the farm
by the spring. dim. Wilt

WADE (AS) (m)–Wanderer
WALTER (T) (m)–Mighty warrior.
dim. Walt
WARD (T) (m)–Guardian
WARREN (T) (m)–Game warden
WAYNE (OE) (m)–A short form of

ZACHARY (m)–A short form of
Zacharia
ZACHARIA (H) (m)–Remembered
by the Lord. var. Zachariah.
dim. Zack, Zach
ZOE (Gr) (f)–Life

In due time—
CONGRATULATIONS!